PREFACE

The purpose of *Pharmacy Calculations* is to provide pharmacy technician students and pharmacy technicians with an educational tool to learn the types of calculations commonly encountered in community and institutional pharmacy. *Pharmacy Calculations* is a solid, basic text that covers topics for everyday practice of pharmacy technicians. Although we initially developed the book as a text for pharmacy technician training programs, the book is also well suited for use by pharmacy technicians working in the field.

The writing provides carefully worded explanations that are direct, easy to understand, and mathematically accurate. The material is presented in a straightforward manner to minimize confusion regarding what pharmacy calculations a technician should know. The format is logical and clear so students can use the book for independent study or as part of a class. Graduates may use this book to review for the pharmacy technician certification exam.

This book allows students to develop a careful and systematic approach to pharmacy calculations. Since pharmacy calculations must be done with 100 percent accuracy, students are encouraged to use a calculator to solve the problems. Students are also invited to practice performing the calculations by hand so they can duplicate their work with 100 percent accuracy.

The second edition of *Pharmacy Calculations* has been revised and expanded based on student and instructor feedback. Chapters 2, 3, 4, 5, and 9 have been updated with new content. Chapter 10 has been enhanced and now includes a section on dimensional analysis, in addition to the section on ratio and proportion, as an approach to solving pharmacy calculations. Chapter 15 includes an additional formula that can be used for temperature conversions. Chapters 16, 17, and 18 have been updated to include dimensional analysis. Chapters 22 and 24 include updated tables for calculating professional fees. Also, more practice problems were added at the end of each chapter.

Introduction

Pharmacy Calculations is divided into three main sections: basic arithmetic, calculations for community pharmacy, and calculations for institutional pharmacy.

- The chapters in Section 1: Basic Arithmetic provide a foundation for the community pharmacy section and the institutional pharmacy section.

- The chapters in Section 2: Calculations for Community Pharmacy include the types of calculations commonly encountered in retail and outpatient settings.

- The chapters in Section 3: Calculations for Institutional Pharmacy include the types of calculations commonly encountered in hospital settings as well as other institutional settings.

The chapters are structured and written as follows:

- The text in each chapter is direct, carefully worded, and concise.

- Each chapter includes a real-world example to show how to work the problems.

- The problems at the end of each chapter are carefully worded and consistent with the material presented in each chapter.

- The number of examples and problems are adequate and appropriate to learn the calculations.

- The way the material is presented allows the student to isolate any chapter in the community pharmacy or institutional pharmacy sections and focus on a specific topic of interest.

- Students are encouraged to use a calculator for routine calculations so they can focus on comprehending and understanding the concepts that are presented.

PHARMACY CALCULATIONS
2ND EDITION

MARY F. POWERS

JANET B. WAKELIN

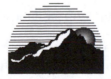

MORTON PUBLISHING COMPANY

925 W. Kenyon Avenue, Unit 12
Englewood, Colorado 80110
www.morton-pub.com

BOOK TEAM

Publisher:	Doug Morton
Project Manager:	Dona Mendoza
Copy Editor:	Kelly Kordes Anton
Cover and Design:	Bob Schram, Bookends
Composition:	International Typesetting & Composition

Printed in the United States of America
by Morton Publishing Company
925 W. Kenyon Ave., Unit 12, Englewood, CO 80110

10 9 8 7 6 5 4 3

ISBN: 0-89582-669-0

ABOUT THE AUTHORS

Mary F. Powers, Ph.D., R.Ph., is Associate Professor of Pharmacy Practice at the University of Toledo College of Pharmacy in Toledo, Ohio. She received her pharmacy degree from the University of Toledo College of Pharmacy and her Doctor of Philosophy in Medical Sciences degree from the Medical College of Ohio, Toledo, Ohio. Powers has extensive experience in community pharmacy practice and has also served as the Pharmacy Technician Program Coordinator at Mercy College of Northwest Ohio, Toledo, Ohio, as an adjunct faculty member at the Medical College of Ohio, and has been involved in teaching pharmacy technicians since 1998.

Janet B. Wakelin, MRPharmS, is the retired Director of the Pharmacy Technician Training Program at Cuyahoga Community College in Cleveland, Ohio. She received her pharmacy degree from Aston University, Birmingham, England. Wakelin has community and hospital experience as a Registered Pharmacist in England and as a Certified Technician in the United States. She served as Treasurer for the Pharmacy Technician Educators Council (PTEC) from 1994 to 1998, and has been involved in teaching pharmacy technicians since 1991. She now lives with her husband in Charlotte, North Carolina.

ACKNOWLEDGMENTS

We want to take this opportunity to thank Doug Morton, whose sponsorship makes this book possible. We also give special thanks to Dona Mendoza, Project Manager at Morton Publishing.

Thank you to Douglas Scribner, Chairman of the Pharmacy Technician Program at Albuquerque Technical Vocational Institute for his suggestions on the initial effort and review of the first edition for errors. Thank you to Dr. Gerhard Lind, Retired Chairman, Department of Chemistry, Metropolitan State College of Denver for his review of the new problems in this second edition for errors. Thank you also to Karen Snipe, Marsha Sanders, and Kim Ballow for their helpful suggestions on the initial effort.

Finally, thank you to supporting colleagues, family, and friends, including: David Wakelin, Ph.D., for checking the institutional math; Nigel Wakelin, Pharm.D. for the chemotherapy examples; Sarah Martin for reading the institutional sections with the eyes of a non-pharmacy person; Mary's dog, Cimmy; Judy Jones-Walker, Ph.D.; Rex and Helen Powers; Sister Joanne Boellner, Ed.D., R.S.M.; and Paul Jomantas.

Sincerely
Mary F. Powers and Janet B. Wakelin

CONTENTS

Answers to Even-numbered Practice Problems 241

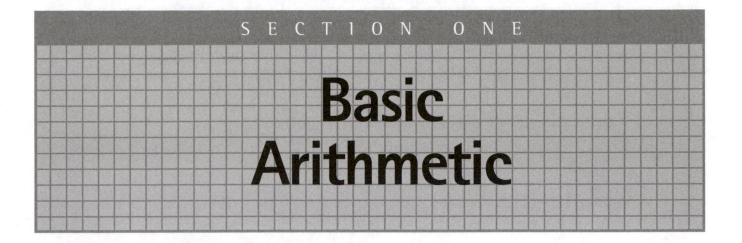

Basic Arithmetic

1 Numeral Systems Used in Pharmacy

ARITHMETIC IS THE BRANCH OF MATHEMATICS in which numbers are used to solve problems. There are many systems in the world for writing numbers. The system for writing numbers that is widely used throughout the world today is based on the number 10 and is known as the Arabic system. In the Arabic system, the position a symbol occupies helps determine the value of the symbol. For example, in 333, the 3 on the right means three, but the 3 in the middle means three tens and the 3 on the left means three hundreds.

Another system for writing numbers that is sometimes used in pharmacy is the Roman numeral system. Roman numerals are expressed by letters of the alphabet and are rarely used today except for formality or variety.

The principles for reading Roman numerals are:

- A letter repeated once or twice repeats its value that many times (XXX = 30, CC = 200, etc.).

- One or more letters that is placed after another letter of greater value increases the greater value by the amount of the smaller (VI = 6, LXX = 70, MCC = 1200, etc.).

- A letter placed before another letter of greater value decreases the greater value by the amount of the smaller (IV = 4, XC = 90, CM = 900, etc.).

The following common Roman numerals correspond to the following values in the Arabic system:

Letter	Value	Letter	Value	Letter	Value	Letter	Value
I	1	VII	7	XL	40	C	100
II	2	VIII	8	L	50	D	500
III	3	IX	9	LX	60	M	1,000
IV	4	X	10	LXX	70		
V	5	XX	20	LXXX	80		
VI	6	XXX	30	XC	90		

Reading Roman numerals requires a different approach than reading Arabic numerals, and generally the position of the Roman numeral is not as important as it is in the Arabic system.

Example:

Convert the Roman numeral XXIX to the Arabic numeral:

XX = 20

IX = 9

XXIX = 20 + 9 = 29

Example:

Convert the Arabic numeral 67 to the Roman numeral:

LX = 60

VII = 7

Combining the two Roman numerals yields: LXVII

P R A C T I C E   P R O B L E M S

STUDENT NAME _____

DATE _____ COURSE NUMBER _____

Convert the following Roman numerals to Arabic numerals:

1. XIX   = _____   11. XXXIII   = _____

2. XC   = _____   12. CIX   = _____

3. CCC   = _____   13. II   = _____

4. XXXII   = _____   14. VIII   = _____

5. XLIV   = _____   15. XXIV   = _____

6. XXII   = _____   16. XXXIV   = _____

7. VII   = _____   17. XLIII   = _____

8. IV   = _____   18. XXVIII   = _____

9. III   = _____   19. XIII   = _____

10. XIX   = _____   20. XXIX   = _____

Convert the following Arabic numerals to Roman numerals:

21. 10   =   _____   31. 4   =   _____

22. 20   =   _____   32. 7   =   _____

23. 30   =   _____   33. 12   =   _____

24. 40   =   _____   34. 16   =   _____

25. 50   =   _____   35. 22   =   _____

26. 15   =   _____   36. 36   =   _____

27. 100   =   _____   37. 49   =   _____

28. 200   =   _____   38. 57   =   _____

29. 300   =   _____   39. 150   =   _____

30. 1,000 =   _____   40. 900   =   _____

2 Numerators, Denominators, and Reciprocals of Fractions

IN THE ARABIC SYSTEM, fractions are used to indicate amounts that fall in between whole numbers. In other words, a fraction represents part of a whole. The division of two whole numbers can also be represented by a fraction. The two parts of a fraction are the numerator and denominator. The denominator (the number below the bar) tells us how many parts the whole is divided into, and the numerator (the number above the bar) tells us how many of those parts exist.

In a fraction, the numerator can be zero, but the denominator cannot be zero. Division by zero is undefined, therefore, no denominator can be zero.

One way to think of a fraction is as division that hasn't been completed yet.

Example:

3/4

You can read this fraction as three-fourths, three over four, or three divided by four.

Fractions can be converted to decimals by performing the division using a calculator:

3/4 = 0.75

Example:

Here are some other fractions and their decimal equivalents. Remember, you can find the decimal equivalent of any fraction by dividing the numerator by the denominator.

2/5 = 0.4
3/5 = 0.6
4/5 = 0.8

There are many ways to write fractions. Fractions that represent the same number are called equivalent fractions. This is basically the same thing as equal ratios. For example, 1/2, 2/4, and 4/8 are all equal. To determine if two fractions are equal, use a calculator and divide. If the answer is the same, then the fractions are equal.

Reciprocals of Fractions

Reciprocals are two different fractions that when multiplied together equals 1. Every fraction has a reciprocal (except those fractions with zero in the numerator). The easiest way to find the reciprocal of a fraction is to switch the numerator and denominator, or just flip the fraction over.

To find the reciprocal of a whole number, just put 1 over the whole number.

Examples:

The reciprocal of 2 is 1/2

The reciprocal of 3 is 1/3

The reciprocal of 4 is 1/4

The reciprocal of 2/3 is 3/2

PRACTICE PROBLEMS

STUDENT NAME _____

DATE _____ COURSE NUMBER _____

Use a calculator to convert the following fractions to decimals:

1.	1/2	=	_____	16.	1/7	=	_____
2.	1/4	=	_____	17.	5/11	=	_____
3.	2/4	=	_____	18.	5/6	=	_____
4.	2/5	=	_____	19.	2/9	=	_____
5.	1/10	=	_____	20.	5/18	=	_____
6.	1/8	=	_____	21.	3/7	=	_____
7.	1/12	=	_____	22.	3/11	=	_____
8.	1/20	=	_____	23.	3/21	=	_____
9.	1/100	=	_____	24.	3/33	=	_____
10.	1/1000	=	_____	25.	5/35	=	_____
11.	3/8	=	_____	26.	7/43	=	_____
12.	3/4	=	_____	27.	9/55	=	_____
13.	4/5	=	_____	28.	13/63	=	_____
14.	1/3	=	_____	29.	15/71	=	_____
15.	7/12	=	_____	30.	23/83	=	_____

Determine the reciprocal of the following fractions:

31.　1/2　　=　_____

32.　1/4　　=　_____

33.　2/4　　=　_____

34.　2/5　　=　_____

35.　1/10　　=　_____

36.　1/8　　=　_____

37.　1/12　　=　_____

38.　1/20　　=　_____

39.　1/100　　=　_____

40.　1/1000　　=　_____

41.　3/8　　=　_____

42.　3/4　　=　_____

43.　4/5　　=　_____

44.　1/3　　=　_____

45.　7/12　　=　_____

46.　1/7　　=　_____

47.　5/11　　=　_____

48.　5/6　　=　_____

49.　2/9　　=　_____

50.　5/18　　=　_____

51.　3/13　　=　_____

52.　3/23　　=　_____

53.　5/7　　=　_____

54.　5/12　　=　_____

55.　5/37　　=　_____

56.　7/48　　=　_____

57.　7/51　　=　_____

58.　9/23　　=　_____

59.　11/52　　=　_____

60.　23/83　　=　_____

3 Reducing Fractions to Lowest Terms

To REDUCE A FRACTION TO LOWEST TERMS, also known as simplifying a fraction, divide the numerator and denominator by their greatest common factor. The greatest common factor is a whole number and both the numerator and denominator can be divided by this number (factor). Some fractions are already in lowest terms if there is no factor common to the numerator and denominator.

The steps to reduce a fraction to its lowest terms are:

1. List the prime factors (a prime factor is a whole number that is divisible by only 1 and itself) of the numerator and denominator.

2. Find the factors common to both the numerator and denominator.

3. Divide the numerator and denominator by all common factors (this is called canceling).

Example:

15/35

1. List the prime factors of the numerator and denominator.

   Numerator: 1,3,5

   Denominator: 1,5,7

2. Divide by, or cancel, the factor of 5 that is common to both the numerator and denominator.

3. You're left with a 3 in the numerator and a 7 in the denominator.

   Numerator: 15/5 = 3

   Denominator: 35/5 = 7

Therefore 15/35 reduced to lowest terms is 3/7.

PRACTICE PROBLEMS

STUDENT NAME _____

DATE _____ COURSE NUMBER _____

Reduce the following fractions to lowest terms:

1.	3/9	= _____	21.	5/11	= _____
2.	6/24	= _____	22.	0/25	= _____
3.	2/4	= _____	23.	75/100	= _____
4.	2/16	= _____	24.	22/55	= _____
5.	6/10	= _____	25.	60/75	= _____
6.	12/36	= _____	26.	30/36	= _____
7.	18/54	= _____	27.	7/28	= _____
8.	10/220	= _____	28.	26/39	= _____
9.	25/125	= _____	29.	27/56	= _____
10.	65/75	= _____	30.	34/51	= _____
11.	21/35	= _____	31.	36/48	= _____
12.	72/90	= _____	32.	24/100	= _____
13.	36/27	= _____	33.	16/32	= _____
14.	15/75	= _____	34.	30/45	= _____
15.	16/24	= _____	35.	28/42	= _____
16.	9/12	= _____	36.	12/35	= _____
17.	6/20	= _____	37.	66/84	= _____
18.	16/40	= _____	38.	14/63	= _____
19.	24/30	= _____	39.	30/70	= _____
20.	14/36	= _____	40.	6/51	= _____

41. 125/500   = _____

42. 25/100   = _____

43. 25/150   = _____

44. 50/500   = _____

45. 270/2700   = _____

46. 65/585   = _____

47. 73/292   = _____

48. 82/164   = _____

49. 79/237   = _____

50. 17/102   = _____

51. 19/285   = _____

52. 18/81   = _____

53. 24/36   = _____

54. 112/280   = _____

55. 59/118   = _____

56. 77/154   = _____

57. 121/605   = _____

58. 63/135   = _____

59. 42/72   = _____

60. 33/77   = _____

4 Adding and Subtracting Fractions

IN ORDER TO ADD OR SUBTRACT FRACTIONS, the fractions must have the same denominator (called common denominators). To add or subtract fractions that have common denominators, you simply add or subtract the numerators and write the sum or difference over the common denominator.

In order to add or subtract fractions with different denominators, you must first find equivalent fractions with common denominators:

1. Find the smallest multiple for the denominator of both numbers.

2. Rewrite the fractions as equivalent fractions with the smallest multiple of both numbers as the denominator.

When working with fractions, the smallest multiple of both denominator numbers is called the least common denominator.

Example:

1/2 + 1/3

The smallest multiple for the denominator of both numbers is 6.

$1/2 = (1 \times 3)/(2 \times 3) = 3/6$

$1/3 = (1 \times 2)/(3 \times 2) = 2/6$

The problem can now be rewritten as:

3/6 + 2/6

Since the denominators are equal, you only need to add the numerators to get the answer.

$(3 + 2)/6 = 5/6$

Example:

4/5 − 1/3

The smallest multiple for the denominator of both numbers is 15.

$4/5 = (4 \times 3)/(5 \times 3) = 12/15$

$1/3 = (1 \times 5)/(3 \times 5) = 5/15$

The problem can now be rewritten as:

12/15 − 5/15

Since the denominators are equal, you only need to subtract the numerators to get the answer.

$(12 − 5)/15 = 7/15$

P R A C T I C E   P R O B L E M S

STUDENT NAME _____

DATE _____ COURSE NUMBER _____

Calculate the following fractions:

1. 1/3 + 1/3 = _____

2. 1/8 + 3/8 = _____

3. 2/3 – 1/3 = _____

4. 5/8 – 3/8 = _____

5. 1/5 + 3/5 = _____

6. 7/8 – 3/8 = _____

7. 1/3 – 1/5 = _____

8. 4/25 + 1/5 = _____

9. 1/8 + 3/16 = _____

10. 7/8 – 1/4 = _____

11. 3/8 + 3/5 = _____

12. 1/5 + 3/5 = _____

13.   2/7   +   3/7   +   1/7   =   _____

14.   4/15   +   6/15   =   _____

15.   1/8   +   2/8   +   7/8   =   _____

16.   1/2   +   3/5   =   _____

17.   3/8   +   11/12   =   _____

18.   5/21   +   5/28   =   _____

19.   2/3   +   1/6   +   5/12   =   _____

20.   5   +   7/10   +   3/1000   =   _____

21.   6/10   –   4/10   =   _____

22.   5/6   –   4/6   =   _____

23.   3/25   +   12/25   =   _____

24.   3/14   –   2/14   =   _____

25.   7/5   –   3/5   =   _____

26.   1/20   +   3/20   =   _____

27.   11/15   –   7/15   =   _____

28.   5/8   +   4/27   +   1/48   =   _____

29.   6   +   1/100   +   3/10   =   _____

30.   1/10   +   3/10   +   9/1000 =   _____

31.   3/5   +   1/5   +   3/10   +   7/10   =   _____

32.   3/4   +   1/4   +   1/8   +   5/8   =   _____

33.   1/12 +   5/12   +   1/3   +   2/3   =   _____

34.   1/9   +   4/9   +   1/3   +   1/18   =   _____

35.   1/2   +   4/5   +   1/10   +   1/20   =   _____

36.   2/9   +   4/9   +   1/2   +   5/18   =   _____

37.   1/7   +   4/7   +   6/35   +   1/35   =   _____

38.   12/19 +   14/38 +   1/19   +   1/38   =   _____

39.   11/12 +   1/3   +   2/3   +   1/24   =   _____

40.   1/5   +   4/5   +   1/10   +   1/20   =   _____

41.   1/2   +   3/4   +   1/3   +   1/12   =   _____

42.   1/3   +   1/4   +   1/12   +   1/24   =   _____

43.   1/2   +   1/3   +   1/4   +   1/24   =   _____

44.   11/99 +   4/9   +   11/33 +   1/18   =   _____

45.   10/90 +   4/9   +   1/3   +   1/18   =   _____

46.   1/8   +   1/4   +   1/2   +   3/8   =   _____

47.   1/3   +   1/6   +   1/9   +   1/18   =   _____

48.   1/2   +   1/9   +   1/36   +   1/18   =   _____

49.   1/5   +   3/10   +   3/20   +   3/40   =   _____

50.   1/19   +   1/38   +   1/76   +   1/152   =   _____

5 Multiplying and Dividing Fractions

Unlike adding and subtracting, when multiplying fractions you do not need a common denominator. To multiply fractions:

1. Multiply the numerators of the fractions to get the new numerator.

2. Multiply the denominators of the fractions to get the new denominator.

3. Simplify the resulting fraction if possible.

Example:

Determine 1/3 of 2/5.

1. Multiply the numerators $(1 \times 2) = 2$.

2. Multiply the denominators $(3 \times 5) = 15$.

3. The resulting fraction is 2/15 (already simplified).

Dividing by fractions is just like multiplying fractions, but there is one additional step to convert the fraction you are dividing by, to its reciprocal. To divide fractions:

1. Find the reciprocal of the fraction you are dividing by.

2. Multiply the first fraction times the reciprocal determined in step 1.

3. Simplify the resulting fraction by reducing to lowest terms, if possible.

Important: Since division by zero is undefined, the number 0 has no reciprocal.

Example:

Divide 24 by 1/4

1. Find the reciprocal of the fraction you are dividing by. The reciprocal of 1/4 is 4/1.

2. Multiply $24/1 \times 4/1 = 96$.

3. Since 96 is a whole number, the answer is already simplified.

Example:

Divide 1/3 by 1/5

1. Find the reciprocal of the fraction you are dividing by. The reciprocal of 1/5 is 5/1.

2. Multiply $1/3 \times 5/1 = 5/3$

3. Simplify 5/3 to 1 2/3.

PRACTICE PROBLEMS

STUDENT NAME_____

DATE _____ COURSE NUMBER _____

Multiply the following fractions:

1.	1/3	of	1/3	=	_____
2.	1/8	of	3/8	=	_____
3.	2/3	of	1/3	=	_____
4.	5/8	of	3/8	=	_____
5.	1/5	of	3/5	=	_____
6.	7/8	of	3/8	=	_____
7.	0/4	of	5/6	=	_____
8.	1/5	of	3/4	=	_____
9.	5/6	of	5/6	=	_____
10.	2/3	of	4/7	=	_____
11.	3/4	of	3/4	=	_____
12.	1/9	of	2/3	=	_____
13.	1/3	×	1/5	=	_____
14.	4/25	×	1/5	=	_____
15.	1/8	×	3/16	=	_____
16.	7/8	×	1/4	=	_____
17.	3/8	×	3/5	=	_____
18.	7/16	×	1/4	=	_____

19. 1/9   ×   4/9   =   _____

20. 2/1   ×   5/1   =   _____

21. 7/10   ×   1/5   =   _____

22. 4/13 ×   2/5   ×   6/7   =   _____

23. 9/100 ×   1   ×   3   =   _____

24. 3/11 ×   0/8   ×   6/7   =   _____

25. 1/3   ×   1/20   ×   1/8   =   _____

26. 1/3   ×   1/4   ×   1/5   ×   3/7   =   _____

27. 4/7   ×   3/5   ×   1/9   ×   1/4   =   _____

28. 1/8   ×   3/8   ×   1/2   ×   1/3   =   _____

29. 3/7   ×   1/2   ×   1/4   ×   1/3   =   _____

30. 5/8   ×   1/3   ×   2/3   ×   3/7   =   _____

31. 3/7   ×   2/7   ×   1/2   ×   1/3   =   _____

32. 1/5   ×   1/3   ×   1/4   ×   1/8   =   _____

33. 3/8   ×   2/3   ×   1/3   ×   3   =   _____

34. 5/8   ×   1/3   ×   1/2   ×   3/8   =   _____

35. 1/9   ×   1/2   ×   1/3   ×   3/7   =   _____

Divide the following fractions:

36. 1/3   divided by   1/3   =   _____

37. 1/8   divided by   3/8   =   _____

38. 2/3   divided by   1/3   =   _____

39. 5/8   divided by   3/8   =   _____

40. 1/5   divided by   3/5   =   _____

41. 7/8   divided by   3/8   =   _____

42.   1/3   divided by   1/5   =   _____

43.   4/25   divided by   1/5   =   _____

44.   1/8   divided by   3/16   =   _____

45.   7/8   divided by   1/4   =   _____

46.   3/8   divided by   3/5   =   _____

47.   3/4   divided by   8/5   =   _____

48.   2/3   divided by   1/2   =   _____

49.   16/27   divided by   8/9   =   _____

50.   5/15   divided by   5   =   _____

51.   9/10   divided by   9/10   =   _____

52.   7/5   divided by   5/7   =   _____

53.   3/5   divided by   0   =   _____

54.   0   divided by   7/8   =   _____

55.   5/24   divided by   3/8   =   _____

56.   7/48   divided by   14/16   =   _____

57.   14/20   divided by   7/4   =   _____

58.   25   divided by   1/5   =   _____

59.   30   divided by   1/10   =   _____

60.   50   divided by   1/2   =   _____

61.   4   divided by   1/2   =   _____

62.   5   divided by   1/5   =   _____

63.   7   divided by   1/14   =   _____

64.   12   divided by   3/8   =   _____

65.   14   divided by   2/7   =   _____

66.   20   divided by   1/10   =   _____

67.   35   divided by   3/10   =   _____

68.   100   divided by   1/3   =   _____

69.   300   divided by   3/8   =   _____

70.   1000   divided by   1/5   =   _____

6 Writing Fractions in Decimal Form

IN THE DECIMAL NUMBER SYSTEM, the value of a digit depends on its place or location in the number. Each place has a value of 10 times the place to its right. Numbers to the left of the decimal point are separated into groups of three digits using commas. As you move right from the decimal point, each place value is divided by 10.

Zero and the counting numbers (1, 2, 3, etc.) make up the set of whole numbers. But not every number is a whole number. The decimal system allows us to write numbers that are fractions as well as whole numbers by using a symbol called the decimal point.

You read the decimal number 105.599 as "one hundred five and five hundred ninety-nine thousandths." The "th" at the end of a word means a fraction part (or a part to the right of the decimal point). You can also read this number as "one hundred five point five nine nine."

Example:

Eight hundred = 800

Eight hundredths = 0.08

Example:

Write the number three hundred twenty-three and four tenths in decimal form:

323.4

Example:

Write the number five hundred fifty-five thousandths in decimal form:

0.555

Example:

Write 13 506/1000 in decimal form:

13.506

PRACTICE PROBLEMS

STUDENT NAME_____

DATE _____ COURSE NUMBER _____

Write the following as decimal numbers:

1. Thirty-two hundredths   = _____
2. Thirty-three thousandths   = _____
3. Two hundred thirty-seven thousandths   = _____
4. Thirty-five and one hundred fifty-three thousandths   = _____
5. Five hundred three and thirty-two hundredths   = _____
6. Eighty-six hundredths   = _____
7. Ninety-nine thousandths   = _____
8. Three tenths   = _____
9. Fourteen thousandths   = _____
10. Seventeen hundredths   = _____
11. Six and twenty-eight hundredths   = _____
12. Sixty and twenty-eight thousandths   = _____
13. Seventy-two and three hundred ninety-two thousandths   = _____
14. Eight hundred fifty and thirty-six ten-thousandths   = _____

Write the following decimal numbers in words:

15. 0.5   =   _____
16. 0.93   =   _____
17. 5.06   =   _____
18. 32.58   =   _____
19. 71.06   =   _____
20. 35.078   =   _____
21. 7.003   =   _____
22. 18.102   =   _____
23. 50.008   =   _____
24. 607.607 =   _____

Write the following decimals as fractions (do not reduce to lowest terms):

25.   593.86   =   _____

26.   0.63   =   _____

27.   0.75   =   _____

28.   0.88   =   _____

29.   0.73   =   _____

30.   0.2   =   _____

31.   0.35   =   _____

32.   0.47   =   _____

33.   0.66   =   _____

34.   0.41   =   _____

35.   0.03   =   _____

36.   1.35   =   _____

37.   3.3   =   _____

38.   4.53   =   _____

39.   6.08   =   _____

40.   10.353   =   _____

41.   20.354   =   _____

42.   31.451   =   _____

43.   49.326   =   _____

44.   51.118   =   _____

45.   101.101   =   _____

7 Rounding Decimals and Significant Figures

SOMETIMES, AFTER MULTIPLYING DECIMAL FRACTIONS or after converting a fraction to a decimal fraction, the number of decimal places is too large to be manageable. Extra numbers can be confusing and can also contribute to errors in calculations. Therefore, it is often useful and advisable to round off decimals.

To round off decimals:

- Find the place value you want (the "rounding digit") and look at the digit just to the right of it.

- If that digit is less than 5, do not change the rounding digit, but drop all digits to the right of it.

- If that digit is greater than or equal to five, add one to the rounding digit and drop all digits to the right of it.

Example:

To round the number 15,732.7343 to the nearest thousandth:

1. Find the rounding digit. This is 4.

2. Look one digit to the right, at the digit in the ten-thousandths place which is "3".

3. See that 3 is less than 5, so leave the number "4," then drop the digits to the right of 4.

This gives 15,732.734.

Example:

To round 622.1352 to the nearest hundredth:

1. Find the rounding digit, "3."

2. Look at the digit one place to right, "5." 5 = 5.

3. Since the rule states if the number to the right of the rounding digit is greater than or equal to 5, add one to the rounding digit and drop all digits to the right of it.

Therefore, this number needs to be rounded up. Add one to the rounding digit and remove all the rest of the digits to the right of it. The result is 622.14

Significant Figures

A significant digit is one that is actually measured. The number of significant digits in a measurement depends on the measuring device used and the sensitivity of that measuring device. When a calculation involves measurements with different numbers of significant figures in the entries or terms that are added, subtracted, multiplied, etc., the answer should have the same number of significant digits as the entry or term with the least number of significant figures in the measurement.

Rules for assigning significant figures:

- Digits other than zero are always significant.

- Final zeros after a decimal point are always significant.

- Zeros between two other significant digits are always significant.

- Zeros used only to space the decimal are never significant.

Example:

Determine the number of significant figures in 3.4502 grams.

Since zeros between two other significant digits are always significant, the number of significant figures is 5.

Example:

Determine the number of significant figures in 3.40 grams.

Since final zeros after a decimal point are always significant, the number of significant figures is 3.

Example:

Determine the number of significant figures in 0.036 grams.

Since zeros used only to space the decimal are never significant, the number of significant figures is 2.

P R A C T I C E   P R O B L E M S

STUDENT NAME _____

DATE _____ COURSE NUMBER _____

Round the following decimal numbers to the nearest hundredth:

1. 132.35789   = _____   6. 2.339   = _____

2. 6.993928394   = _____   7. 1.006   = _____

3. 2.357895733   = _____   8. 3.232323232   = _____

4. 235,121.34764   = _____   9. 101.234   = _____

5. 132,424,324.351   = _____   10. 136.567   = _____

Round off each decimal number to the nearest tenth:

11. 80.015   = _____   16. 0.037   = _____

12. 7.555   = _____   17. 3.2323   = _____

13. 180.009   = _____   18. 44.444   = _____

14. 37.6666   = _____   19. 365.365   = _____

15. 14.3332   = _____   20. 0.245   = _____

Round off each decimal number to the nearest whole number:

21. 32.134   = _____   27. 2.95   = _____

22. 55.556   = _____   28. 3.25   = _____

23. 109.421   = _____   29. 145.2   = _____

24. 0.76   = _____   30. 3.33   = _____

25. 100   = _____   31. 4.12   = _____

26. 1.00   = _____   32. 54.329   = _____

33.	100.01	=	_____	37.	512.8	=	_____
34.	325.2	=	_____	38.	1000.9	=	_____
35.	467.1	=	_____	39.	2001.09	=	_____
36.	479.9	=	_____	40.	345.59	=	_____

Determine the number of significant figures in each measurement:

41. 6.222 g   =   _____

42. 0.123 kg   =   _____

43. 12.0 ml   =   _____

44. 0.030 g   =   _____

45. 20.05 grams   =   _____

8 Adding and Subtracting Decimal Numbers

Adding and subtracting decimals is just like adding and subtracting whole numbers. When adding and subtracting decimals, it is very important to line up the terms so that all the decimal points are in a vertical line.

To add decimal numbers:

1. Put the numbers in a vertical column, aligning the decimal points.

2. Add each column of digits, starting on the right and working left. If the sum of a column is more than 10, "carry" the digits to the next column on the left.

3. Place the decimal point in the answer directly below the decimal points in the terms.

Example:

Step 1:

```
   324.5678
+    1.2345
─────────────
          3 (carry the 1)
```

Step 2:

```
   324.5678
+    1.2345
─────────────
         23 (carry the 1)
```

Step 3:

```
   324.5678
+    1.2345
─────────────
        023 (carry the 1)
```

Step 4:

```
   324.5678
+    1.2345
─────────────
       .8023
```

Step 5:

```
   324.5678
+    1.2345
─────────────
      5.8023
```

Step 6:

```
   324.5678
+    1.2345
─────────────
     25.8023
```

Step 7:

```
   324.5678
+    1.2345
─────────────
    325.8023
```

To subtract decimal numbers:

1. Put the numbers in a vertical column, aligning the decimal points.

2. Subtract each column, starting on the right and working left. If the digit being subtracted in a column is larger than the digit above it, "borrow" a digit from the next column to the left.

3. Place the decimal point in the answer directly below the decimal points in the terms.

Example

Step 1:

```
   32.255
 −  1.203
         2
```

Step 2:

```
   32.255
 −  1.203
        52
```

Step 3:

```
   32.255
 −  1.203
      .052
```

Step 4:

```
   32.255
 −  1.203
     1.052
```

Step 5:

```
   32.255
 −  1.203
    31.052
```

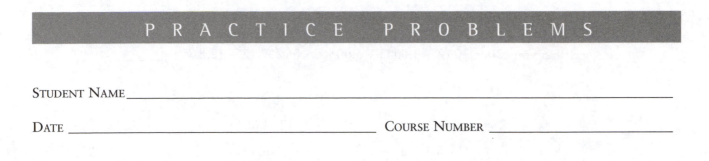

PRACTICE PROBLEMS

STUDENT NAME _____

DATE _____ COURSE NUMBER _____

Add the following decimal fractions:

1. 0.6 + 0.4 + 1.3 = _____

2. 5 + 6.1 + 0.4 = _____

3. 0.59 + 6.91 + 0.05 = _____

4. 3.488 + 16.593 + 25.002 = _____

5. 37.02 + 25 + 6.4 + 3.89 = _____

6. 4.0086 + 0.034 + 0.6 + 0.05 = _____

7. 43.766 + 9.33 + 17 + 206 = _____

8. 52.3 + 6 + 21.01 + 4.005 = _____

9. 2.0051 + 0.2006 + 5.4 + 37 = _____

10. 5 + 2.37 + 463 + 10.88 = _____

11. 2 + 3 + 3.5 + 4.6 + 5.5 = _____

12. 2.4 + 1.3 + 1.5 + 4.3 + 15.9 = _____

13. 1.1 + 2.2 + 3.3 + 4.4 + 5.5 = _____

14. 12 + 3.5 + 3.3 + 144 + 155 = _____

15. 20 + 30 + 4.55555 + 400.6 + 501.5 = _____

16. 2.2 + 3.3 + 5.5 + 6.6 + 7.5 + 7.7 = _____

17. 122 + 301 + 55.5 + 6.5 + 701.5 + 7.007 = _____

18. 2 + 3 + 5 + 6.6663 + 7.501 + 12.0007 = _____

19. $12.2 + 23.3 + 55.5 + 36.6 + 7.0005 + 7.7 = $ _____

20. $212 + 3.0003 + 5.005 + 6.06 + 7.12 + 12.8 = $ _____

21.   22.   23.

      354.2312   224.0021   5223.2312
 +   5.1092   +   6.4444   +   65.3217

24.   25.

   22375.23   34.2312875
 +   5.92   + 22.1092

Subtract the following decimal fractons:

26. $5.2 - 3.76$ =   _____   36. $3.8 - 2.12$ =   _____

27. $17.83 - 8.9$ =   _____   37. $5 - 0.002$ =   _____

28. $29.5 - 13.61$ =   _____   38. $13.01 - 12$ =   _____

29. $1.0057 - 0.03$ =   _____   39. $123 - 0.001$ =   _____

30. $78.015 - 13.068$ =   _____   40. $117.2 - 117$ =   _____

31. $22.418 - 17.524$ =   _____   41. $145.45 - 0.44$ =   _____

32. $4.8 - 0.0026$ =   _____   42. $136.3 - 125.2$ =   _____

33. $31.009 - 0.534$ =   _____   43. $111 - 0.01$ =   _____

34. $4 - 1.0566$ =   _____   44. $110 - 0.1$ =   _____

35. $40.718 - 6.532$ =   _____   45. $345.34 - 1.32$ =   _____

46.

354.2312
−   5.1092
――――――

47.

224.0012
−   6.4444
――――――

48.

5223.2312
−   65.3217
――――――

49.

22375.23
−   5.92
――――――

50.

34.2312875
− 22.1092
――――――

9 Multiplying Decimal Numbers

MULTIPLICATION IS OFTEN INDICATED by an "×" inserted between numbers. Another way to indicate multiplication is to separate adjacent numbers by parentheses. Multiplication can also be indicated by a "·" or "*" that is inserted between numbers.

To multiply decimal numbers:

1. Multiply the numbers just as if they were whole numbers.

2. Line up the numbers on the right (do not align the decimal points).

3. Starting on the right, multiply each digit in the top number by each digit in the bottom number

4. Add the products.

5. Place the decimal point in the answer by starting at the right and moving the point the number of places equal to the sum of the decimal places in both numbers that were multiplied together.

6. Line up the numbers on the right in the same way you would if there were no decimal points.

7. Start at the right side and multiply each digit in the top number by each digit in the bottom number.

8. Add the product resulting from multiplying each digit of the bottom number.

9. Place the decimal point in the answer so that the number of decimal places in the answer equals the total number of decimal places in both numbers that were multiplied together.

Example:

47.2×5.5:

```
     47.2 (has 1 decimal place)
×     5.5 (has 1 decimal place)
   ─────
    2360
+  2360
   ─────
  259.60 (2 decimal places)
```

Example:

Find the product of 9.683×6.1:

```
     9.683 (has 3 decimal places)
×      6.1 (has 1 decimal place)
    ──────
     9683
+  58098
    ──────
   59.0663 (3 + 1 = 4 decimal places)
```

PRACTICE PROBLEMS

STUDENT NAME _____

DATE _____ COURSE NUMBER _____

Multiply the following decimals:

1.	(0.6)(0.7)	=	_____	21.	122.1(212.12)	=	_____
2.	(0.3)(0.8)	=	_____	22.	3.3 * 4.4	=	_____
3.	(0.2)(0.2)	=	_____	23.	5.52 * 4.1	=	_____
4.	(0.3)(0.3)	=	_____	24.	3.741 * 2.122	=	_____
5.	8(2.7)	=	_____	25.	15.41 * 12.12	=	_____
6.	4(9.6)	=	_____	26.	144.44 * 2.3	=	_____
7.	1.4(0.3)	=	_____	27.	513.312 * 0.5	=	_____
8.	1.5(0.6)	=	_____	28.	25.12 * 0.2	=	_____
9.	(0.2)(0.02)	=	_____	29.	12.2 * 0.3	=	_____
10.	(0.3)(0.03)	=	_____	30.	36.63 * 1.5	=	_____
11.	5.4(0.02)	=	_____	31.	122 * 4.2	=	_____
12.	7.3(0.01)	=	_____	32.	42.24 *42.24	=	_____
13.	0.23(0.12)	=	_____	33.	135.1 * 10	=	_____
14.	(0.15)(0.15)	=	_____	34.	146.63 * 100	=	_____
15.	(8.1)(0.006)	=	_____	35.	1.235 * 1,000	=	_____
16.	7.1(0.008)	=	_____	36.	4.222 * 0.01	=	_____
17.	0.06(0.01)	=	_____	37.	31.31 * 13.1	=	_____
18.	0.25(0.01)	=	_____	38.	10 * 0.1	=	_____
19.	(3.23)(2.32)	=	_____	39.	100 * 0.01	=	_____
20.	14.5(15.4)	=	_____				

40.
$$\begin{array}{r} 35.23 \\ \times\ \ 22.12 \\ \hline \end{array}$$

41.
$$\begin{array}{r} 253.424 \\ \times\ \ \ \ \ 4.2 \\ \hline \end{array}$$

42.
$$\begin{array}{r} 2.5 \\ \times\ \ 3.27 \\ \hline \end{array}$$

43.
$$\begin{array}{r} 527.225 \\ \times\ \ \ \ 2.1 \\ \hline \end{array}$$

44.
$$\begin{array}{r} 2.38795 \\ \times\ \ \ \ \ \ 1.1 \\ \hline \end{array}$$

45.
$$\begin{array}{r} 326.311 \\ \times\ \ 2.113 \\ \hline \end{array}$$

46.
$$\begin{array}{r} 1.21 \\ \times\ \ 3.333 \\ \hline \end{array}$$

10 Using Ratios and Proportions or Dimensional Analysis to Solve Pharmacy Calculations

MOST CALCULATIONS IN PHARMACY can be solved using either of two techniques: ratio and proportion or dimensional analysis.

Ratio and Proportion

Ratios are used to make comparisons between two things. When you express ratios in words, you use the word "to." For example, you say "the ratio of something to something else."

A ratio can be written in several different ways: as a fraction, using the word "to," or with a colon.

Example:

The following expressions all represent the ratio "3 to 5":

3/5

3 to 5

3:5

Equal ratios are two different ratios that may include different numbers when expressed as fractions, but can be reduced to the same fraction. To find an equal ratio, multiply or divide each term in the ratio by the same number (but not zero).

Example:

If you divide both terms in the ratio 3:6 by the number three, then you get the equal ratio, 1:2. Examples of other equal ratios include:

3:6 = 12:24 = 6:12 = 15:30

These can also be expressed as:

3/6 = 12/24 = 6/12 = 15/30

Proportions

A proportion is a name given to a statement that two ratios are equal. Proportions can be written in two ways:

- As two equal fractions, a/b = c/d

- Using a colon, a:b = c:d

When two ratios are equal, then the products of the means (or middle numbers) equals the products of the extremes (or outside numbers).

Example:

For the proportion a:b = c:d , b × c (means) = a × d (extremes)

The proportion 20/30 = 2/3 is read as "twenty is to thirty as two is to three."

In problems involving proportions, you can test the products of the means and extremes to test whether two ratios are equal and form a proportion.

The ratios 20/30 and 2/3 form a proportion because the product of the means equals the product of the extremes.

$30 \times 2 = 60$

$20 \times 3 = 60$

Dimensional Analysis

Dimensional analysis is a useful method scientists employ to check the validity of scientific equations and calculations. For some very complicated problems in science, sometimes, dimensional analysis is the only way to find the right answer! Dimensional analysis can also be used for most pharmacy calculations either to check your work, or, once you've mastered the technique, may be the best way to get the correct answer to your problem. Some people find dimensional analysis to be extremely helpful for complicated pharmaceutical calculations.

In science, the dimension of an object tells you what sort of quantity it is. In science, there are four basic dimensions: length, mass, time, and electrical charge. Similarly, in pharmacy we can think of pharmaceutical quantities in terms of the "dimensions" such as weight, volume, dose, dosage form, and time (day[s]).

To solve a problem using dimensional analysis, you need to first identify what information is provided by the problem as well any conversion factors that you will need to solve the problem. Terms that are equal to each other are written in the form of a fraction. For example, if 250 mg = 1 dose, you would write this as a fraction

$$\frac{250 \text{ mg}}{1 \text{ dose}} \quad \text{or} \quad \frac{1 \text{ dose}}{250 \text{ mg}}$$

Since both fractions are equal to 1, you can write either term in the numerator. Once you have written all of the information, you need to solve the problem in the form of fractions. To do this, you simply setup a series of fractions (making sure to label each term!) in an equation so that when the fractions are multiplied, all units will cancel out, except the units you need for your answer.

Example:

You can use dimensional analysis to determine how many capsules are needed to fill a prescription for amoxicillin 250 mg/capsule, one capsule three times per day for seven days:

Use dimensional analysis to solve this problem:

$$\frac{capsule}{250 \ mg} \times \frac{250 \ mg}{dose} \times \frac{3 \ doses}{day} \times 7 \ days = 21 \ capsules$$

1. Start by setting up a dimensional analysis equation so the units you want in the final answer (the capsule) is in the numerator of the first fraction of the dimensional analysis equation.

2. Set up the next fraction in the dimensional analysis equation so the units of the numerator of the second fraction are the same as the units of the denominator of the first fraction (that is, so the units cancel when the fractions are multiplied).

3. Set up the next fraction in the dimensional analysis equation so the units of the numerator of the third fraction are the same as the units of the denominator of the second fraction (again, so the units cancel when the fractions are multiplied).

4. Set up the next fraction in the dimensional analysis equation so the units of the numerator of the fourth fraction are the same as the units of the denominator of the third fraction (again, so the units cancel when the fractions are multiplied).

5. Multiply the fractions!

Important: Always remember to check your work!

For this example, when all fractions are multiplied together, all units cancel except the capsule units (which is in the numerator). When using dimensional analysis, you need to be careful to make sure that the numerator (not the denominator) contains the units you need to solve the problem.

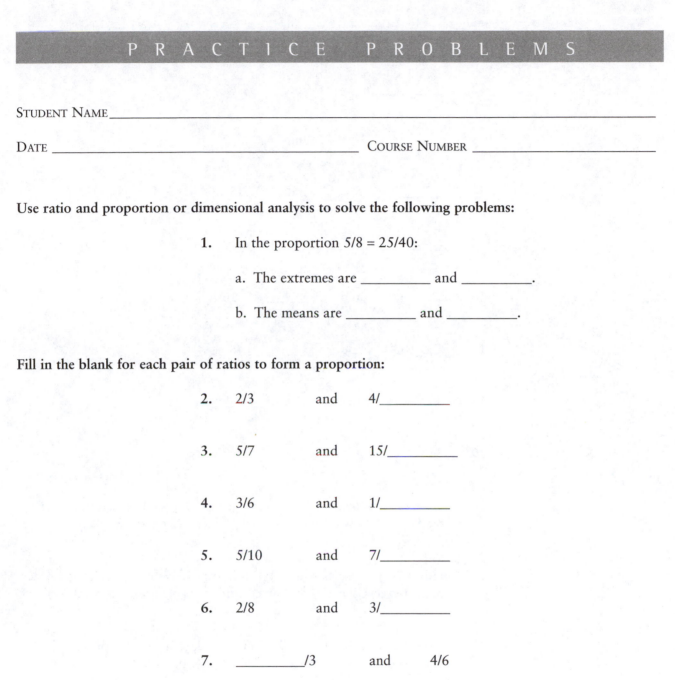

PRACTICE PROBLEMS

STUDENT NAME_____

DATE _____ COURSE NUMBER _____

Use ratio and proportion or dimensional analysis to solve the following problems:

1. In the proportion 5/8 = 25/40:

    a. The extremes are _____ and _____.

    b. The means are _____ and _____.

Fill in the blank for each pair of ratios to form a proportion:

2. 2/3   and   4/_____

3. 5/7   and   15/_____

4. 3/6   and   1/_____

5. 5/10   and   7/_____

6. 2/8   and   3/_____

7. _____/3   and   4/6

8. _____/8   and   3/24

9. _____/12   and   5/6

10. _____/4   and   6/8

11.   _____/5   and   10/25

12.   _____/6   and   10/12

13.   _____/7   and   6/42

14.   _____/15   and   2/5

15.   _____/5   and   4/10

16.   3/5   and   _____/100

17.   125/1000   and   _____/8

18.   3/8   and   375/_____

19.   2/3   and   _____/12

20.   How many tablets will be taken in seven days if a prescription order reads zafirlukast 20 mg/tablet, one tablet twice a day?

21.   How many capsules will be taken in three days if a prescription order reads tetracycline 250 mg/capsule, one capsule four times a day?

22.   How many tablets will be taken in five days if a prescription order reads sucralfate 1 g/tablet, one tablet four times a day?

23.   How many tablets will be taken in 10 days if a prescription order reads zaleplon 5 mg/tablet, one tablet daily at bedtime?

24.   How many tablets will be taken in 30 days if a prescription order reads methylphenidate 10 mg/tablet, one tablet three times a day?

25.   How many capsules are needed to fill a prescription for 30 days for zidovudine 100 mg/capsules, three capsules twice daily?

26.   How many tablets are needed to fill a prescription for 34 days for nabumetone 500 mg/tablet, one tablet twice daily?

27.   How many tablets will be taken in 10 days if a prescription order reads metoclopramide 5 mg/tablet, one tablet three times a day?

28.   How many tablets will be taken in 10 days if a prescription order reads rabeprazole 20 mg/tablet, one tablet twice a day?

29.   How many tablets will be taken in seven days if a prescription order reads albuterol 2 mg/tablet, one tablet four times a day?

30.   How many tablets will be taken in two days if a prescription order reads promethazine 12.5 mg/tablet, one tablet three times a day?

31.   How many tablets will be taken in five days if a prescription order reads fluphenazine 1 mg/tablet, one tablet three times a day?

32.   How many capsules are needed to fill a prescription for 14 days for ampicillin 500 mg/capsule, one capsule four times a day?

33.   How many tablets are needed to fill a prescription for 30 days for primadone 250 mg/tablet, one tablet three times a day?

34.   How many tablets are needed to fill a prescription for 34 days for acarbose 50 mg/tablet, one tablet three times a day?

35.   How many capsules are needed to fill a prescription for 34 days for prazosin 1 mg/capsules, two capsules three times a day?

36.   How many tablets are needed to fill a prescription for 21 days for repaglinide 0.5 mg/tablet, one tablet three times a day?

37.   How many capsules are needed to fill a prescription for 34 days for potassium chloride 10 mEq/capsule, one capsule four times a day?

38.   How many capsules are needed to fill a prescription for three days for mefenamic acid 250 mg/capsule, one capsule four times a day?

39.   How many tablets are needed to fill a prescription for 21 days for dipyridamole 50 mg/tablet, one tablet four times a day?

40.   How many tablets are needed to fill a prescription for seven days for cyproheptadine 4 mg/tablet, one tablet three times a day?

11 Percents

THE TERM "PERCENT" means "per 100" or "out of 100."

The percent symbol (%) can be used as a way to write a fraction with a common denominator of 100.

Example:

20 out of every 100 equals 20%

Example:

5 out of every 100 equals 5%

Example:

15% = 15/100 = 0.15

Fifteen percent (15%) is the same as the fraction 15/100 and the decimal 0.15.

You can write percents as decimals by moving the decimal point two places to the left.

You can also write decimals as percents, by moving the decimal point two places to the right.

Example:

Express 27% as a decimal.

Since you can write a percent as a decimal by moving the decimal point two places to the left:

27% = 0.27

Example:

Express 0.85 as a percent.

Since you can write decimals as percents by moving the decimal point two places to the right:

.85 = 85%

Example:

Calculate 30% of 300.

1. Change 30% to a decimal by moving the decimal point two places to the left: 30% = 0.30
2. Then multiply: $0.30 \times 300 = 90$

Therefore, 30% of 300 is 90.

Example:

Write 6 out of 12 as a percent.

6 out of 12 = 0.5 = 50%

Example:

Find the value of n if n is 50% of 60.

n = 0.5 × 60 = 30

Example:

Find the value of n if n is 150% of 24.

n = 1.5 × 24 = 36

PRACTICE PROBLEMS

STUDENT NAME _____

DATE _____ COURSE NUMBER _____

Express the following percents as decimals:

1.	33%	=	_____	9.	75%	=	_____
2.	24%	=	_____	10.	83.32%	=	_____
3.	33.3%	=	_____	11.	66.66667%	=	_____
4.	50.5%	=	_____	12.	18.5%	=	_____
5.	20%	=	_____	13.	1.3%	=	_____
6.	47%	=	_____	14.	0.25%	=	_____
7.	93%	=	_____	15.	0.125%	=	_____
8.	32.5%	=	_____				

Express the following decimals as percents:

16.	0.2444	=	_____	26.	0.52	=	_____
17.	0.3	=	_____	27.	0.4	=	_____
18.	0.5	=	_____	28.	0.65	=	_____
19.	0.125	=	_____	29.	0.025	=	_____
20.	0.75	=	_____	30.	0.035	=	_____
21.	0.02	=	_____	31.	0.055	=	_____
22.	0.09	=	_____	32.	0.004	=	_____
23.	0.1	=	_____	33.	1.10	=	_____
24.	0.8	=	_____	34.	1.75	=	_____
25.	0.36	=	_____	35.	2	=	_____

Calculate the following:

36.   25% of 600   =   _____   44.   110% of 5   =   _____

37.   20% of 30   =   _____   45.   33% of 90   =   _____

38.   15% of 20   =   _____   46.   5% of 50   =   _____

39.   75% of 50   =   _____   47.   30% of 120   =   _____

40.   12.5% of 24   =   _____   48.   40% of 50   =   _____

41.   80% of 40   =   _____   49.   60% of 150   =   _____

42.   90% of 100   =   _____   50.   70% of 400   =   _____

43.   17% of 10   =   _____

Write the following expressions as percents:

51.   4 out of 5   =   _____   59.   6 out of 20   =   _____

52.   2 out of 10   =   _____   60.   12 out of 20   =   _____

53.   7 out of 8   =   _____   61.   35 out of 40   =   _____

54.   15 out of 20   =   _____   62.   40 out of 50   =   _____

55.   30 out of 35   =   _____   63.   55 out of 100   =   _____

56.   85 out of 100   =   _____   64.   80 out of 90   =   _____

57.   5 out of 8   =   _____   65.   32 out of 64   =   _____

58.   3 out of 7   =   _____

Find the value of n:

66.   If n is 20% of 50   n =   _____   71.   If n is 40% of 30   n =   _____

67.   If n is 35% of 24   n =   _____   72.   If n is 50% of 100   n =   _____

68.   If n is 60% of 8   n =   _____   73.   If n is 25% of 50   n =   _____

69.   If n is 75% of 10   n =   _____   74.   If n is 30% of 90   n =   _____

70.   If n is 80% of 15   n =   _____   75.   If n is 100% of 50   n =   _____

12 Exponents and Scientific Notation

EXPONENTS ARE A SHORTHAND WAY to show how many times a number is multiplied times itself. A number with an exponent is said to be "raised to the power" of that exponent.

Example:

$3^4 = 3 \times 3 \times 3 \times 3 = 81$

Any number raised to the zero power (except 0) equals 1.

Example:

$3^0 = 1$

Any number raised to the power of one equals itself.

Example:

$3^1 = 3$

Scientific Notation

Scientific notation is a short way of writing very long numbers. On a calculator, scientific notation is also known as E notation ("E" stands for "Exponent").

A number written in scientific notation is written as a product of a number between 1 and 10 and a power of 10.

Example:

Write 438,680,000 in scientific notation.

1. Change the number to a number between 1 and 10 by moving the decimal point 8 places to the left.

2. Multiply by 10 raised to the power of the number of places you had to move the decimal point.

$438,680,000 = 4.3868 \times 10^8$

On a calculator window, the base of 10 is not shown; the E means "10 raised to the following power."

Example:

Write the following numbers in scientific notation.

$434,000 = 4.34 \times 10^5$

$8,421,000 = 8.421 \times 10^6$

$23,412,000,000 = 2.3412 \times 10^{10}$

P R A C T I C E P R O B L E M S

STUDENT NAME _____

DATE _____ COURSE NUMBER _____

Express the following as numbers:

1. 2^3 = _____

2. 1^0 = _____

3. 1^1 = _____

4. 10^3 = _____

5. 3^{10} = _____

6. 6^6 = _____

7. 12^3 = _____

8. 10^5 = _____

9. 4^4 = _____

10. 5^5 = _____

11. 3^2 = _____

12. 4^3 = _____

13. 6^4 = _____

14. 7^2 = _____

15. 9^2 = _____

16. 10^2 = _____

17. 3^4 = _____

18. 4^7 = _____

19. 5^2 = _____

20. 6^3 = _____

Write the following numbers in scientific notation:

21.   12   = _____   31.   100   = _____

22.   456   = _____   32.   1,000   = _____

23.   5,309   = _____   33.   5   = _____

24.   78,322   = _____   34.   15   = _____

25.   104,043   = _____   35.   30   = _____

26.   1,567,334   = _____   36.   6,100   = _____

27.   0.12   = _____   37.   712   = _____

28.   0.125   = _____   38.   503   = _____

29.   0.0056   = _____   39.   35   = _____

30. 2^3 = _____   40.   1,000,000 = _____

13 Converting Household and Metric Measurements

THE METRIC SYSTEM IS WIDELY USED in medicine. The strength of a medication is almost always given in metric units, most commonly the milligram (mg). For example, atenolol 50 mg tablets have 50 mg of the active ingredient (atenolol) in each tablet; however, if you weighed each tablet on a scale, you would find each tablet weighs much more than 50 mg (due to binders and fillers that are needed for the tablet to take form and hold together).

The metric system was developed in the late 1700s to replace a system with illogical units of measure with a rational system based on multiples of 10. The meter is the standard unit of length in the metric system and the length of the meter is based on the arc of the meridian from Barcelona, Spain, to Dunkirk, France. All metric units were derived from the meter. The gram is the standard measure of weight in the metric system (which is the weight of one cubic centimeter (cc) of water at its maximum density).

Greek prefixes were established for multiples of 10, ranging from pico- (one-trillionth) to tera- (one trillion) and including the more familiar micro- (one-millionth), milli- (one-thousandth), centi- (one-hundredth), and kilo- (one thousand). Thus, a kilogram equals 1,000 grams, a millimeter 1/1,000 of a meter.

One cubic centimeter (cc) is equal to one milliliter (ml). A milliliter is a measure of volume and there are 1,000 milliliters in one liter.

Factor	Name	Symbol
10^9	giga	G
10^6	mega	M
10^3	kilo	k
10^2	hecto	h
10^1	deka	da
10^{-1}	deci	d
10^{-2}	centi	c
10^{-3}	milli	m
10^{-6}	micro	μ
10^{-9}	nano	n
10^{-12}	pico	p

Example:

How many centimeters (cm) are in one meter?

Since the prefix centi means 10^{-2}, there are 10^2 (or 100) centimeters in one meter.

Example:

How many milliliters (ml) are in one liter?

Since the prefix milli means 10^{-3}, there are 10^3 (or 1,000) milliliters in one liter.

Converting Measurements

Medications are prepared by drug manufacturers according to the metric standards and measurements used in science. Pharmacies have an important duty to accurately convert metric measurements for the dose of medication to household measurements to ensure that patients get the correct dose of medication. The pharmacy label should provide information so the patient can read the directions on the prescription bottle, measure the correct dose of medication, and take the correct dose of medication.

Liquid medications taken by mouth are commonly dispensed in community pharmacies. Some but not all measuring spoons and measuring cups are labeled with both household and metric units. The directions are usually printed on the prescription label so the volume can be measured using household measuring devices such as measuring spoons, cups, etc.

Household Measure	Metric Equivalent
1 teaspoonful (tsp.)	5 ml
1 tablespoonful (Tbl.)	15 ml
1 fluid ounce (fl. oz.)	29.6 ml (often rounded to 30 ml)
1 pint (pt.)	473 ml (often rounded to 480 ml)
1 gallon (gal.)	3785 ml
1 pound (lb.)	454 gm

The conversions between household and metric measurements can be done by carefully setting up proportions as fractions, then multiplying the fractions to get the correct answer.

Important: Always be sure you are using the correct conversion factors when setting up ratio and proportion or dimensional analysis equations.

Example:

Convert 2 tsp. to ml.

1. Start by setting up a dimensional analysis equation so the units you want in the final answer are in the numerator of the first fraction. 5 ml/1 tsp.

2. Set up the next fraction so the units of the numerator in the second fraction are the same as the units of the denominator in the first fraction (that is, so the units cancel when the fractions are multiplied). 2 tsp.

3. Multiply the fractions! Always be sure the numerator contains the units of the measuring device that you are using for your measurement. 5 ml/1 tsp. × 2 tsp. = 10 ml.

Important: Always double check your work to be sure the units cancel and the numerator contains the correct units. Also, be sure there was not an error using the calculator!

5 ml/1 tsp. × 2 tsp. = 10 ml

Common Pharmacy Abbreviations

Abbreviations are commonly used in prescriptions to provide information that is necessary to prepare and administer the medication.

a.c.	before food
ad	to, up to
ad lib.	freely
bib.	drink
b.i.d.	twice a day
c̄	with
gt or gtt	drop
h.s.	at bedtime
i.m.	into the muscle
i.v.	into the vein
non rep. or nr	do not repeat
o.d.	right eye
o.s.	left eye
o.u.	both eyes
p.c.	after food
p.o.	by mouth
p.r.	by rectum
p.r.n.	as needed
qAM	each morning
q.d.	each day
q.h.	each hour
q[2,3,4...]h	every [two, three, four, etc.] hours
q.i.d.	four times a day
Rx	take
s̄	without
s.l.	under the tongue
stat.	immediately
t.i.d.	three times a day

Example:

If a prescription reads: 7.5 ml t.i.d., what is the dose in household units?

1 tsp./5 ml × 7.5 ml/dose = 1.5 tsp./dose

1. Start by setting up a dimensional analysis equation so the units you want in the final answer are in the numerator of the first fraction. 1 tsp./5 ml

2. Set up the next fraction so the units of the numerator in the second fraction are the same as the units of the denominator in the first fraction (that is, so the units cancel when the fractions are multiplied). 7.5 ml/dose

3. Multiply the fractions! Always be sure the numerator contains the units of the measuring device that you are using for your measurement. 1 tsp./5 ml × 7.5 ml/dose = 1.5 tsp./dose

Important: Again, remember to check your work!

Example:

If a prescription reads: Amoxicillin 250 mg/5ml, dispense 150 ml, 375 mg t.i.d. × 5d, what is the dose in household units?

1 tsp./5 ml × 5 ml/250 mg × 375 mg/dose = 1.5 tsp./dose

Example:

If a medication is ordered 5mg/kg/day and is administered once daily, what is the dose for a 150-pound patient?

5 mg/kg/day × kg/1000 gm × 454 gm/lb × 150 lb = 340.5 mg/day

PRACTICE PROBLEMS

STUDENT NAME_____

DATE _____ COURSE NUMBER _____

Convert the following:

1. 1/3 tsp.   = _____ ml

2. 3 tsp.   = _____ ml

3. 2 pints   = _____ ml

4. 1/2 lb.   = _____ gm

5. 3 quarts   = _____ ml

6. 1/2 tsp.   = _____ ml

7. 11/2 tsp.   = _____ ml

8. 3 gal.   = _____ ml

9. 3 tablespoonsful = _____ ml

10. 2 fl. oz.   = _____ ml

11. 3 fl. oz.   = _____ ml

12. 3 pints   = _____ ml

13. 3 lbs.   = _____ gm

14. ml   = _____ tsp.

15. 45 ml   = _____ fl. oz.

16. 15 ml   = _____ tsp.   = _____ Tbl.

17. 2,365 ml   = _____ pints

18. 22,710 ml   = _____ gal.

19. 2 ml   = _____ tsp.

20.   20 ml   =   _____ tsp.

21.   908 gm   =   _____ lbs.

22.   45 ml   =   _____ tsp.

23.   100 gm   =   _____ lbs.

24.   3 Tbl.   =   _____ ml

25.   5 fl. oz.   =   _____ ml

26.   5 lbs.   =   _____ kg

27.   1,135 gm   =   _____ lbs.

28.   2 pt.   =   _____ ml

29.   473 ml   =   _____ pt.

30.   0.9 kg   =   _____ lbs.

31.   9,080 gm   =   _____ lbs.

32.   1,000 mg   =   _____ gm

33.   0.908 kg   =   _____ lbs.

34.   3.785 liters   =   _____ gal.

35.   1.816 kg   =   _____ lbs.

36.   1.75 tsp.   =   _____ ml

37.   7.5 ml   =   _____ Tbl.

38.   30 ml   =   _____ tsp.

39.   60 ml   =   _____ Tbl.

40.   88.8 ml   =   _____ fl. oz.

41. If a prescription reads: Cefaclor 250 mg/5ml, dispense 150 ml, 375 mg b.i.d. × 10d, what is the dose in teaspoonsful?

42. If a prescription reads: Erythromycin 200 mg/5ml, 200 mg t.i.d. × 5d, what is the dose in teaspoonsful?

43. If the dose of a medication is 30 mg/kg/day in four divided doses, what is each dose for a 205-pound patient?

44. If a prescription reads: Amoxicillin 50 mg/ml, dispense 30 ml, 62.5 mg t.i.d. × 5d, what is the dose in teaspoonsful?

45. How many gallons of Coca Cola fountain syrup are needed to package 144 bottles of 120 ml per bottle?

14 Converting Apothecary and Metric Measurements

SOME PRESCRIBERS ORDER MEDICATIONS using the apothecary system of measurement. The most commonly used apothecary measures are grains (to measure weight of solids) and drams (to measure volume of liquids).

Apothecary Measures

Apothecary Measure	Metric Equivalent
1 grain	64.8 mg (often rounded to 65 mg)
1 dram	5 ml
1 fl. oz.	29.6 ml (often rounded to 30 ml)
1 oz. (apothecary)	31 gm

You can also perform the conversions between apothecary and household measurements by carefully setting up proportions as fractions, then multiplying the fractions to get the correct answer.

Important: Always be sure you are using the correct conversion factor when setting up ratio and proportion or dimensional analysis equations. Always double check your calculations!

Example:

Convert 129.6 mg to grains.

gr./64.8 mg × 129.6 mg = 2 gr.

Example:

If a prescription reads: Amoxicillin 250 mg/5ml, dispense 150 ml, 1 dram t.i.d. × 10d, what is the dose in household units?

1 tsp./5 ml × 5 ml/1 dram × 1 dram/dose = 1 tsp./dose

Example:

If a prescription reads: aspirin 5 gr, dispense 100 tablets, 1 tablet q4-6h prn headache, what is the dose in milligrams?

64.8 mg/grain × 5 grains/tablet × 1 tablet/dose = 324 mg/dose

Important: Always be sure you are using the correct conversion factor when setting up ratio and proportions or dimensional analysis equations, and always double check your calculations!

STUDENT NAME_____

DATE _____ COURSE NUMBER _____

Convert the following:

1.	3 gr.	=	_____	mg
2.	1/2 gr.	=	_____	mg
3.	3 drams	=	_____	fl. oz.
4.	3 drams	=	_____	ml
5.	1/2 dram	=	_____	ml
6.	120 mg	=	_____	gr.
7.	2 oz. (apothecary)	=	_____	gm
8.	20 ml	=	_____	drams
9.	30 ml	=	_____	drams
10.	4 fl. oz.	=	_____	ml
11.	1/4 grain	=	_____	mg
12.	2 drams	=	_____	ml
13.	3 fl. oz.	=	_____	ml
14.	6 oz. (apothecary)	=	_____	gm
15.	2 grains	=	_____	mg
16.	5 drams	=	_____	ml
17.	2 fl. oz.	=	_____	ml
18.	12 oz. (apothecary)	=	_____	gm
19.	97.2 mg	=	_____	grains

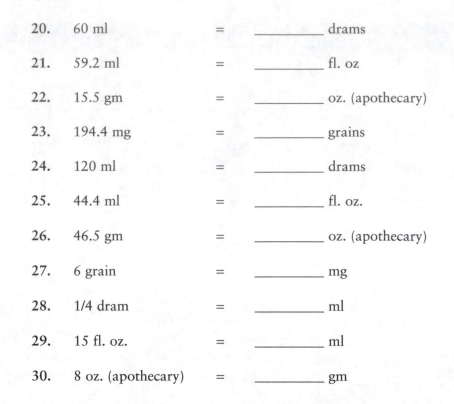

20.   60 ml   =   _____ drams

21.   59.2 ml   =   _____ fl. oz

22.   15.5 gm   =   _____ oz. (apothecary)

23.   194.4 mg   =   _____ grains

24.   120 ml   =   _____ drams

25.   44.4 ml   =   _____ fl. oz.

26.   46.5 gm   =   _____ oz. (apothecary)

27.   6 grain   =   _____ mg

28.   1/4 dram   =   _____ ml

29.   15 fl. oz.   =   _____ ml

30.   8 oz. (apothecary) =   _____ gm

31.   If a prescription reads: Amoxicillin 250 mg/5ml, dispense 150 ml, 1 dram t.i.d. × 10d, what is the dose in teaspoonsful?

32.   How many mg of phenobarbital are in one tablet of 2 grain phenobarbital?

33.   How many doses are in a 100 ml bottle of penicillin VK 250 mg/5 ml if each dose is 1/2 teaspoonful?

34.   If 100 tablets contain 40,000 mg of ibuprofen, how many grains are in 500 tablets?

35.   If a prescription reads: Theophylline Elixir 80 mg/15 ml, what is the dose in teaspoonsful if the required dose is 120 mg?

15 Converting Between the Different Temperature Scales

The temperature for storing medication is extremely important for the stability—and hence effectiveness—of the medication. The two common temperature scales used in pharmacy are Celsius and Fahrenheit. Usually storage requirements (including storage temperature) are listed in small print on the package label. The necessary temperature is usually given in both Celsius and Fahrenheit degrees, although not always. Therefore, you need to be able to convert between Celsius and Fahrenheit.

To convert to degrees Celsius from degrees Fahrenheit, use the following formula:

Tc = (5/9)*(Tf – 32); Tc = temperature in degrees Celsius, Tf = temperature in degrees Fahrenheit

(In the formula, / means to divide, * means to multiply, – means subtract, + means to add and = means equals.)

Example:

Convert the Fahrenheit temperature of 98.6 degrees into degrees Celsius.

Using the above formula, first subtract 32 from the Fahrenheit temperature and get 66.6. Then, you multiply 66.6 by 5/9 and get 37 degrees Celsius.

The formula to convert a Celsius temperature into degrees Fahrenheit is:

Tf = (9/5)*Tc + 32; Tc = temperature in degrees Celsius, Tf = temperature in degrees Fahrenheit

(In the formula, / means to divide, * means to multiply, – means subtract, + means to add and = means equals.)

Example:

Convert the Celsius temperature of 100 degrees into degrees Fahrenheit.

Using the preceeding formula, you first multiply the Celsius temperature reading by 9/5 and get 180. Then, you add 32 to 180 and get 212 degrees Fahrenheit.

The temperature conversion formula can be simplified to:

9C = 5F – 160

Some people find the formula 9C = 5F – 160 is easier to use.

Example:

Use the formula 9C = 5F – 160 to convert the Celsius temperature of 100 degrees into Fahrenheit.

9(100) = 5F – 160

900 + 160 = 5F

1060 = 5F

212 = F

PRACTICE PROBLEMS

STUDENT NAME _____

DATE _____ COURSE NUMBER _____

Convert the following:

1. 25 degrees Celsius = _____ degrees Fahrenheit

2. 15 degrees Celsius = _____ degrees Fahrenheit

3. 30 degrees Celsius = _____ degrees Fahrenheit

4. 45 degrees Celsius = _____ degrees Fahrenheit

5. 10 degrees Celsius = _____ degrees Fahrenheit

6. 20 degrees Celsius = _____ degrees Fahrenheit

7. 5 degrees Celsius = _____ degrees Fahrenheit

8. 30 degrees Celsius = _____ degrees Fahrenheit

9. 40 degrees Celsius = _____ degrees Fahrenheit

10. 50 degrees Celsius = _____ degrees Fahrenheit

11. 22 degrees Celsius = _____ degrees Fahrenheit

12. 32 degrees Celsius = _____ degrees Fahrenheit

13. 47 degrees Celsius = _____ degrees Fahrenheit

14. 2 degrees Celsius = _____ degrees Fahrenheit

15. 12 degrees Celsius = _____ degrees Fahrenheit

16. −5 degrees Celsius = _____ degrees Fahrenheit

17. −10 degrees Celsius = _____ degrees Fahrenheit

18. 7 degrees Celsius = _____ degrees Fahrenheit

19. 37 degrees Celsius = _____ degrees Fahrenheit

20.   18 degrees Celsius   =   _____ degrees Fahrenheit

21.   90 degrees Fahrenheit   =   _____ degrees Celsius

22.   70 degrees Fahrenheit   =   _____ degrees Celsius

23.   32 degrees Fahrenheit   =   _____ degrees Celsius

24.   15 degrees Fahrenheit   =   _____ degrees Celsius

25.   80 degrees Fahrenheit   =   _____ degrees Celsius

26.   75 degrees Fahrenheit   =   _____ degrees Celsius

27.   60 degrees Fahrenheit   =   _____ degrees Celsius

28.   25 degrees Fahrenheit   =   _____ degrees Celsius

29.   55 degrees Fahrenheit   =   _____ degrees Celsius

30.   100 degrees Fahrenheit   =   _____ degrees Celsius

31.   5 degrees Fahrenheit   =   _____ degrees Celsius

32.   12 degrees Fahrenheit   =   _____ degrees Celsius

33.   22 degrees Fahrenheit   =   _____ degrees Celsius

34.   37 degrees Fahrenheit   =   _____ degrees Celsius

35.   45 degrees Fahrenheit   =   _____ degrees Celsius

36.   58 degrees Fahrenheit   =   _____ degrees Celsius

37.   63 degrees Fahrenheit   =   _____ degrees Celsius

38.   79 degrees Fahrenheit   =   _____ degrees Celsius

39.   82 degrees Fahrenheit   =   _____ degrees Celsius

40.   89 degrees Fahrenheit   =   _____ degrees Celsius

Calculations for Community Pharmacy

16 Calculations for Compounding

COMPOUNDS ARE PREPARED in pharmacies for prescription orders that are not commercially available in the strength or form needed. Careful calculations are necessary to be sure the patient receives the proper dose of medication. You can also perform these calculations by carefully setting up ratio and proportion or dimensional analysis equations.

Important: Always be sure you are using the correct conversion factor when setting up ratio and proportion or dimensional analysis equations. Always double check your calculations!

Example:

How much hydrocortisone and how much Eucerin Cream must be weighed out to prepare the following compound?

Hydrocortisone 2.5% in Eucerin Cream
Dispense 60 gm
Sig: Apply sparingly b.i.d. prn

1. Calculate how much hydrocortisone is needed:

    2.5 gm HC/100 gm total × 60 gm total = 1.5 gm HC

2. Calculate how much Eucerin cream is needed:

    Total weight = weight of hydrocortisone + weight of Eucerin cream

    Using algebra, you can solve for the weight of the Eucerin cream:

    Weight of Eucerin cream = Total weight − weight of hydrocortisone

    Weight of Eucerin cream = 60 gm − 1.5 gm = 58.5 gm

Example:

If 100 gm of salicylic acid ointment contains 20 grams of salicylic acid, what is the percent strength of salicylic acid in the ointment?

20 gm salicylic acid/100 gm total ointment = 0.20 = 20%.

Reconstitution of Liquid Antibiotics for Oral Use

Most liquid antibiotics for oral use are shipped from the manufacturer in a powder form for reconstitution. Distilled water is usually used for reconstitution of oral liquid antibiotics. In the powder form, the medications have a longer shelf life than the liquid forms. Also, the powder forms can usually be stored at room temperature. After reconstitution (adding the distilled water), the liquid antibiotics must often be stored in the refrigerator and their shelf life is limited (usually 10 days to 35 days). Information about the shelf life of the reconstituted drug and also how much distilled water must be added to get the desired concentration is printed on the manufacturer's label.

Frequently, the manufacturer suggests that you add the distilled water in two-steps, so the liquid antibiotic is not lumpy. Lumpy liquid antibiotics do not have uniform concentration of drug, and this can lead to variability in dosing.

Example:

To reconstitute a 150 ml bottle of amoxicillin for oral suspension 250 mg/5 ml, the manufacturer recommends 88 ml of distilled water is added in two divided portions. First, loosen the powder in the bottle, then add approximately 1/3 of the total volume of water and shake the suspension. After the powder is wet, add the remaining water. How much water should you add each time?

The first step is to calculate 1/3 of the total volume:

1/3 × 88 ml = 29.3 ml

The second step is to calculate the remaining amount of water:

Total volume = volume of 1st addition + volume of 2nd addition

Volume of 2nd addition = total volume − volume of 1st addition = 88 ml − 29 ml = 59 ml

PRACTICE PROBLEMS

STUDENT NAME_____

DATE _____ COURSE NUMBER _____

1. How much clindamycin phosphate (150 mg/ml) and how much
    Cetaphil Lotion are needed to prepare the following compound?

    Clindamycin phosphate 600 mg in Cetaphil Lotion
    Dispense 60 ml
    Sig: Apply hs ud

2. A prescription is written for equal parts hydrocortisone cream 2.5%
    and Lamisil Cream, dispense 30 gm. How many grams of
    hydrocortisone 2.5% cream is needed to fill this prescription?
    What is the final concentration of hydrocortisone in the compound?

3. A prescription is written for: Acyclovir 1200 mg, Silica gel.
    micronized 0.12 gm, Polyethylene glycol 3350 6.5 gm, Polyethylene
    glycol 400 15 ml. How many 200 mg capsules of acyclovir are needed
    to prepare this compound?

4. A prescription is written for Allopurinol liquid 20 mg/ml in
    Ora-Plus:Ora-Sweet 1:1 (label with a shelf-life of 60 days). How
    many tablets of allopurinol 100 mg are needed to prepare 150 ml?

5. A prescription is written for Dilantin 5% in zinc oxide qs 120 gm. How
    many Dilantin 50 mg tablets are needed to prepare this compound?

6. A prescription is written for ibuprofen 10% cream. How much
    ibuprofen powder is needed to prepare 30 grams of this compound?

7.   A prescription is written for Ichthammol Ointment 2 oz. How much ichthammol is needed to prepare 2 oz. if you are using the following formula: 100 grams of Ichthammol, 100 grams of Lanolin, 800 grams of Petrolatum, to make 1000 grams.

8.   A prescription is written for levothyroxine Na 25 mcg/ml, 100 ml to be compounded from crushed triturated with glycerin 40 ml (levitating agent and rinse for mortar and pestle) and water (q.s. 100 ml). This compound is stable for eight days when stored at 4 deg C. in amber bottles. How many 0.1 mg levothyroxine tablets are needed to prepare this compound?

9.   A prescription is written for Metoprolol tartrate 10 mg/ml Oral Liquid in a 50:50 mixture of Ora-Sweet:Ora Plus Vehicle q.s. 120 ml. How many Metoprolol tartrate 100 mg tablets are needed to prepare this compound?

10.   A prescription is written for Tetracycline HCl suspension 125 mg/5 ml compounded from capsules and a mixture of Ora-Plus 50% and Ora-Sweet 50%. How many capsules of Tetracycline 250 mg are needed to prepare 100 ml of this suspension?

11.   A prescription is written for salicylic acid 1%, menthol 1/4% in triamcinolone 0.1% cream. How much salicylic acid powder should be used if the prescription is for 240 gm?

12.   A prescription is written for a mouthwash containing 170 ml diphenhydramine elixir, 50 ml lidocaine viscous, 200 ml nystatin suspension, 52 ml of erythromycin ethyl succinate suspension, and 28 ml of cherry syrup to make 500 ml mouthwash. How much lidocaine viscous would be needed if you only need to prepare 100 ml of the mouthwash?

13.   You need to prepare 100 ml of hydrocortisone 2 mg/ml suspension. How many hydrocortisone 20 mg tablets will you need?

14.   You need to prepare 70 ml of lansoprazole 3 mg/ml suspension. How many lansoprazole 30 mg capsules will you need?

15.   You need to prepare 120 ml of potassium bromide 250 mg/ml. How much potassium bromide should you weigh?

16.   You need to prepare 150 ml of clonidine 0.1 mg/5 ml suspension. How many tablets of clonidine 0.2 mg/tablet will you need?

17.   You need to prepare 300 ml of methylphenidate 10 mg/5 ml suspension. How many tablets of methylphenidate 20 mg/tablet will you need?

18.   You need to prepare 50 ml of captopril 1 mg/ml suspension. How many tablets of captopril 50 mg/tablet will you need?

19.   You need to prepare 45 ml of baclofen 10 mg/ml. How many tablets of baclofen 10 mg/tablet will you need?

20.   You need to prepare 15 ml of amiptriptyline 20 mg/ml suspension. How many tablets of amitriptyline 50 mg/tablet will you need?

21.   You need to prepare 90 ml of hydrochlorothiazide 10 mg/ml. How many tablets of hydrochlorothiazide 25 mg/tablet will you need?

22. You need to prepare 30 gm of salicylic acid 40% in petrolatum. How many gm of salicylic acid will you need?

23. You need to prepare 150 ml of metformin 100 mg/ml suspension. How many tablets of metformin 500 mg/tablet will you need?

24. You need to prepare a 150 ml of metronidazole 59 mg/5 ml suspension. How many tablets of metronidazole 250 mg/tablet will you need?

25. You need to prepare 60 ml of enalapril 1 mg/ml suspension. How many tablets of enalapril 10 mg/tablet will you need?

26. You need to prepare 120 ml of amiodarone 5 mg/ml suspension. How many tablets of amiodarone 200 mg/tablet will you need?

27. You are preparing hydrocortisone 2.4 g in 240 ml Lubriderm lotion. What is the percent strength of the hydrocortisone?

28. You need to prepare 100 ml of celecoxib 100 mg/5 ml. How many capsules of 200 mg celecoxib/capsule will you need?

29. You need 408 mg of promethazine to prepare 240 ml of PAC syrup. How many ml of promethazine 50 mg/ml will you need?

30. You need to prepare 10 ml nitroglycerin 0.1 mg/ml from a stock vial of nitroglycerin 5 mg/ml diluted with normal saline. What volume of nitroglycerin 5 mg/ml will you need?

17 Calculations for Days Supply

INSURERS AND OTHER THIRD PARTIES that pay some or all of the price of a prescription have guidelines or dispensing limitations for how many days worth of medication they will pay for in a given time frame. The most common days supply limitation by third-party plans is a 34-day supply, although other days supply limitations exist, such as 30-day, 21-day, 14-day, etc.

Most prescribers write prescriptions with a different time frame in mind. Common prescribing time frames include 5 days, 1 week, 2 weeks, 1 month, 50 days, or 100 days.

Days Supply of Tablets, Liquids, Creams, Insulin, Inhalers, Eye Drops

Calculations for days supply should be the best estimate of how long a medication should last if it is used properly.

You can also use ratio and proportion or dimensional analysis to solve calculations for days supply.

Example:

A prescription is written for Amoxicillin 250 mg capsules #30 i cap t.i.d. What is the days supply?

30 capsules × day/3 capsules = 10 days

Example:

A prescription is written for Amoxicillin 250 mg/5 ml 150 ml i tsp. t.i.d. What is the days supply?

150 ml × tsp./5 ml × dose/1 tsp. × day/3 doses = 10 days

Example:

A prescription is written for Mycolog II cream 15 gm apply sparingly twice a day. What is the days supply?

Calculations for creams are a little more tricky because you usually don't know how much cream will be used in a dose. The amount will depend on how large of an area is affected. The amount applied usually does not exceed 500 mg to 1 gram, so unless you know otherwise, use 1 gram for the amount of the dose.

15 gm × dose/1 gm × day/2 doses = 7.5 days (can round to 8 days)

Example:

A prescription is written for Humulin N U-100 insulin 10 ml 35 units daily. What is the days supply?

10 ml × 100 units/ml × dose/35 units × day/1 dose = 28.57 days (can round to 29 days)

Example:

A prescription is written for Albuterol Inhaler 17 gm 2 puffs q.i.d. What is the days supply?

To solve this problem, you should first read the manufacturer's label on the Albuterol Inhaler to determine how many metered doses are in each 17 gm container.

After reading the label, you determine each 17 gm container delivers 200 metered doses and you have enough information to solve the problem.

200 doses/1 container × day/8 doses = 25 days

Example:

A prescription is written for Timolol 0.25% Opth.Sol. 5 ml i gtt ou q.d. What is the days supply?

To solve this problem you need to know how many drops are in 1 ml. The number of drops per ml is not a constant number and varies depending on physical properties of the solution or suspension as well as the size of the hole in the dropper. For most solutions or suspensions, there are 15–20 drops per ml. For the purpose of calculating days supply for third party claims, you can use 20 drops = 1 ml; however, this is only an estimation and *cannot* be used to calculate dosage.

5 ml/bottle × 20 drops/ml × day/2 drops = 50 days

Some medications, such as methylprednisolone, come in handy convenience packages or dosage packages. For these types of medication, you can make a good estimate of the days supply if you have the package in your hand and can visually examine how it is packaged and read from the labeling or package insert how long the contents of the package should last.

PRACTICE PROBLEMS

STUDENT NAME_____

DATE _____ COURSE NUMBER _____

Calculate days supply for the following prescriptions:

1.	Zantac 150 mg #60 one b.i.d.	_____ days
2.	Augmentin 500 mg #42 one t.i.d.	_____ days
3.	Prilosec 20 mg #50 one q.d.	_____ days
4.	Ampicillin 500 mg #40 one q.i.d.	_____ days
5.	Prozac 20 mg #60 one q.d.	_____ days
6.	Lamisil Cream 15 gm apply daily	_____ days
7.	Premarin 0.625 mg #100 one q.d. days 1-25	_____ days
8.	Z-Pak 500 mg PO on first day of therapy, then 250 mg PO once daily for 4 days. Total cumulative dose 1.5 g	_____ days
9.	Tylenol #3 Disp. #30 one-two q4-6h prn pain	_____ days
10.	Xanax 0.25 mg #30 one t.i.d. prn	_____ days
11.	Terazol-7 Cream 45 gm Insert 1 applicatorful (5 gm) hs × 7d	_____ days
12.	Lac-Hydrin 12% Lotion 150 ml Apply lotion twice daily to the affected skin areas and rub in thoroughly. (Hint: use 1–2 ml for amount used per application unless you know a larger area is being treated.)	_____ days
13.	MetroGel Vaginal Gel 70 gm One applicatorful (37.5 mg of metronidazole/5 g cream) intravaginally b.i.d. × 5D	_____ days

14.   Nizoral Cream 15 gm
      Apply to the affected and surrounding areas once
      daily for 2 weeks   _____ days

15.   Bactroban Oint. 15 gm
      Apply a small amount to the affected area t.i.d.
      × 1–2 weeks   _____ days

16.   Humulin N U-100 10 ml
      35 U SQ daily   _____ days

17.   Celebrex 200 mg #25
      1 cap q.d.   _____ days

18.   Ultram 50 mg #20
      1–2 tab q4-6h prn pain   _____ days

19.   Flonase 16 gm
      2 sprays per nostril (1 spray = 50 µg)
      once daily for a total daily dose of 200 µg   _____ days

20.   Neosporin Opth. Ointment 3.5 gm
      Apply a thin strip (approx. = 1 cm ou
      q3-4 h × 7-10 d (Hint: 100 mg per eye per
      application is a useful estimate.)   _____ days

21.   Ortho-TriCyclen 28
      One qd   _____ days

22.   Viagra 50 mg #3
      50 mg PO prn
      not to exceed once daily   _____ days

23.   Vioxx 25 mg/5 ml 150 ml
      12.5 mg q.d.   _____ days

24.   Medrol Dosepak (#21 tablets)
      Take as labeled
      (Hint: see package, package insert or reference
      book for packaging information.)   _____ days

25.   Tobradex Opth. Susp. 5 ml
      Instill 1–2 drops into the conjunctival sac
      os q4-6h   _____ days

26.   Atrovent Inhalation Solution 0.02%
      2.5 ml × 25 vials
      1 vial q.i.d.   _____ days

27. Vanceril Inhaler 17 gm
     2 sprays (42 µg/spray) p.o. q.i.d.   _____ days

28. If a prescription is written for ibuprofen 600 mg, i tab q.i.d., what is
     the maximum quantity allowed if the third party plan has a 21-day
     dispensing limitation?

29. Atenolol 50 mg #100
     One q.d.   _____ days

30. Amoxicillin 250 mg #30
     One q8h   _____ days

31. Lisinopril 10 mg #30
     One daily   _____ days

32. Hydrochlorothiazide 25 mg #30
     One q.d.   _____ days

33. Furosemide Oral 20 mg po #25
     One q.d.   _____ days

34. Alprazolam 0.5 mg #30
     One t.i.d.   _____ days

35. Cephalexin 250 mg #28
     One q6h   _____ days

36. Propoxyphene-N/APAP N-100 #60
     One q.i.d.   _____ days

37. Metformin 500 mg #60
     One b.i.d.   _____ days

38. Fluoxetine 20 mg #40
     One q.d.   _____ days

39. Metoprolol Tartrate 50 mg #60
     One b.i.d.   _____ days

40. Potassium Chloride 10 mEq #60
     One b.i.d.   _____ days

41. Amoxicillin/Pot Clav 250 mg chewable #30
     One t.i.d.   _____ days

42. Ranitidine HCl 150 mg #60
     One b.i.d.   _____ days

43.   Amitriptyline 25 mg #30
      One h.s.   _____ days

44.   Trimethoprim/Sulfa DS #20
      One b.i.d.   _____ days

45.   Cyclobenzaprine 10 mg #30
      One t.i.d.   _____ days

46.   Penicillin VK 500 mg #28
      One q.i.d.   _____ days

47.   Tramadol 50 mg #36
      One q.i.d.   _____ days

48.   Carisoprodol 350 mg #40
      One q.i.d.   _____ days

49.   Verapamil SR 240 mg #30
      One q.d.   _____ days

18 Adjusting Refills for Short–filled Prescriptions

T HE AMOUNT OF MEDICATION a pharmacy can dispense to a patient is restricted first, by the prescriber's guidelines and second by the insurer's guidelines. Calculations are often needed to adjust first the quantity dispensed to comply with the insurer's guidelines, and then the number of refills allowed. Pharmacy technicians often need to accurately estimate how long a medication will last with inadequate guidelines. Estimating days supply is especially tricky when the dosage form is a lotion, cream, ointment, or inhalant.

When dispensing medications that come in handy convenience packages or dosage packages, such as methylprednisolone, estimate the days supply when you have the package in your hand so you can visually examine how it is packaged and read from the labeling or package insert how long the contents of the package should last. Usually, it is inappropriate to disrupt the packaging for medications that come in convenience packages or dosage packages.

Example:

A prescription is written for Dyazide #50 i cap q.d. + 3 refills. The insurance plan has a 34-day supply limitation. How many capsules can be dispensed using the insurance plan guidelines and how many refills are allowed with the adjusted quantity?

1. Calculate the total number of capsules allowed by the prescriber

   50 capsules × 4 total fills (original fill + 3 refills) = 200 capsules

2. Using dimensional analysis, calculate the total number of fills of 34 capsules allowed:

   200 capsules × fill/34 capsules = 5.88 fills

The original prescription will have 4 additional refills of 34 capsules + 1 partial refill of 30 capsules.

Example:

A prescription is written for Rondec-DM Syrup 1 pint 1 teaspoonful h.s. + 1 refill. The insurance plan has a 34-day supply limitation. How many ml can be dispensed using the insurance plan guidelines and how many refills are allowed with the adjusted quantity?

1. Calculate the total volume allowed by the prescriber.

   1 pint × 2 fills (1 + 1 refill) = 2 pints

2. Convert to the metric quantity.

   2 pints × 473 ml/1 pint = 946 ml

3. Calculate the volume for a 34-day supply.

   5 ml/dose × 1 dose/day × 34 days/bottle = 170 ml

4. Calculate the number of refills.

   946 ml total × fill/170 ml = 5.56 total fills

Therefore, the answer is an original fill of 170 ml + 4 refills of 170 ml + a partial refill.

To calculate the amount of the partial refill:

.56 × 170 ml = 96 ml

You can check this:

946 ml − (5 fills × 170 ml per fill = 850 ml) = 96 ml

PRACTICE PROBLEMS

STUDENT NAME_____

DATE _____ COURSE NUMBER _____

Calculate the amount per fill allowable if a third-party plan covers a 34-day supply and adjust the refills:

1.   Nitrolingual Pumpspray #3
     (200 sprays/container)
     1–2 metered doses (400–800 μg)
     SL. May repeat q5 minutes up to a max.
     × 3 doses/15 min
     2 refills

     _____ qty   _____ refills   _____ partial

2.   Atrovent Inhalation Solution 0.02%
     2.5 ml × 25 vials dispense 10 boxes
     1 vial q.i.d
     2 refills

     _____ qty   _____ refills   _____ partial

3.   Humulin N U-100 Insulin 10 ml
     Dispense 4 bottles
     20 units daily
     3 refills

     _____ qty   _____ refills   _____ partial

4.   Ultram 50 mg #120
     1 b.i.d.
     1 refill

     _____ qty   _____ refills   _____ partial

5.   Timoptic 0.25% 10 ml
     Dispense 2 bottles
     1 gtt ou q.d.
     3 refills

     _____ qty   _____ refills   _____ partial

6. Betoptic 0.5% 10 ml
Dispense 2 bottles
1 gtt ou b.i.d.
3 refills

_____ qty   _____ refills   _____ partial

7. Tobradex Opth. Susp. 5 ml
1 gtt od q3-4h
1 refill

_____ qty   _____ refills   _____ partial

8. Gentamicin Sulfate Opth. Ung. 3.5 gm
Apply os b.i.d.
1 refill

_____ qty   _____ refills   _____ partial

9. MS Contin 30 mg #120
1 b.i.d.
No refill

_____ qty   _____ refills   _____ partial

10. Cardizem CD 240 mg #120
1 q.d.
1 refill

_____ qty   _____ refills   _____ partial

11. Amitriptyline 25 mg #100
1 h.s.
1 refill

_____qty   _____refills   _____ partial

12. Methocarbamol 500 mg #240
1000 mg p.o. q.i.d.
1 refill

_____qty   _____refills   _____ partial

13. Nabumetone 500 mg #100
1 g p.o. q.d.
2 refills

_____qty   _____refills   _____ partial

14. Dicyclomine 20 mg #200
20 mg p.o .q.i.d.
1 refill

_____qty   _____refills   _____ partial

15.   Chlorhexidine Glucon 500 ml
       15 ml swish for 30 sec then spit b.i.d.
       3 refills

       _____qty   _____refills   _____ partial

16.   Albuterol Oral Liq 2mg/5 ml 1 pint
       2 mg p.o. t.i.d.
       1 refill

       _____qty   _____refills   _____ partial

17.   Carbamazepine 200 mg #200
       1 q.i.d.
       2 refills

       _____qty   _____refills   _____ partial

18.   Indomethacin 25 mg #100
       1 b.i.d.
       2 refills

       _____qty   _____refills   _____ partial

19.   hydroxychloroquine 200 mg #100
       2 q.d.
       2 refills

       _____qty   _____refills   _____ partial

20.   Digoxin 0.125 mg #100
       1 q.d.
       3 refills

       _____qty   _____refills   _____ partial

21.   Doxepin 150 mg #100
       One q.d. h.s.
       No refill

       _____qty   _____refills   _____ partial

22.   Mirtazapine 15 mg #50
       One q.d. h.s.
       No refill

       _____qty   _____refills   _____ partial

23.   Amiodarone 200 mg #100
       One q.d.
       No refill

       _____qty   _____refills   _____ partial

24. Baclofen 20 mg #120
     One t.i.d.
     1 refill

     _____qty   _____refills   _____ partial

25. Benztropine 1 mg #100
     One b.i.d.
     1 refill

     _____qty   _____refills   _____ partial

26. Indapamide 1.25 mg #100
     One q.d.
     1 refill

     _____qty   _____refills   _____ partial

27. Labetalol 200 mg #100
     One b.i.d.
     1 refill

     _____qty   _____refills   _____ partial

28. Diltiazem SR 120 mg #100
     One b.i.d.
     2 refills

     _____qty   _____refills   _____ partial

29. Carbidopa/Levodopa 25/250 #100
     One b.i.d.
     2 refills

     _____qty   _____refills   _____ partial

30. Etodolac 400 mg #200
     One t.i.d.
     2 refills

     _____qty   _____refills   _____ partial

19 Calculations for Dispensing Fees, Co-pays, Difference Pricing

DISPENSING FEES ARE FEES that are determined by a contractual agreement between the third party and the pharmacy to pay for the expenses associated with dispensing each prescription (labor, equipment, rent, packaging, labeling, etc.).

Co-pays are determined by a contractual agreement between the third party and the patient and are usually determined by the insurer and/or employer providing the prescription drug benefits. Most co-pays are fixed dollar amounts and vary if a brand name or generic medication are dispensed. Some co-pays reflect a percent of the cost of the medication.

Example:

What is the co-pay for a prescription of Amoxicillin 250 mg #30 if the co-pay is 20% of the usual and customary price for the prescription and the usual and customary price for Amoxicillin 250 mg #30 is $8.49?

$0.2 \times \$8.49 = \$1.70$

Some insurance plans specify difference pricing must be used to calculate the co-pay of a prescription when a generic is available, but sometimes the patient refuses to get the generic. Although pharmacy technicians do not usually calculate difference pricing; it is helpful to understand difference pricing. The mathematical formula used to calculate the difference price varies among different third party plans and is specified in a contractual agreement. The difference price is usually determined by the sum of the co-pay amount plus the difference in cost between the brand and generic medication.

Example:

What is the co-pay for a prescription of Motrin 400 mg #20 if the brand name is specified by the patient, the co-pay amount is $5, the cost of Motrin 400 mg #20 is $3.74 and the cost of ibuprofen 400 mg #20 is $2.22?

$5	+	($3.74 − $2.22 = $1.52)	=	$6.52
standard		difference in cost between		difference
co-pay		brand and generic		price co-pay

Example:

How much will a pharmacy be reimbursed for a prescription if the third-party contract states the pharmacy will be reimbursed at 85% of AWP + $2.50 dispensing fee, and if the AWP for the prescription is $23.65?

0.85	× $23.65	= $20.10 +	$2.50	= $22.60
(fraction equal to 85%)	AWP		dispensing fee	amount pharmacy is reimbursed

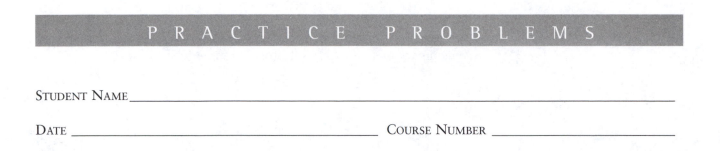

STUDENT NAME_____

DATE _____ COURSE NUMBER _____

Determine the following copays if difference pricing is required by the third party plan.

1. What is the co-pay for a prescription of Hydrochlorothiazide 25 mg
    #30 if the co-pay is $5 and the usual and customary price for
    Hydrochlorothiazide 25 mg #30 is $6.09?

2. What is the co-pay for a prescription of Micronase 5 mg #30 if the
    brand name is specified by the patient, the co-pay amount is $7, the
    cost of Micronase 5 mg #30 is $12.74, and the cost of Glyburide
    5 mg #30 is $4.08?

3. What is the co-pay for a prescription of Deltasone 5 mg #20 if the
    brand name is specified by the patient, the co-pay amount is $3, the
    cost of Deltasone 5 mg #20 is $2.08, and the cost of prednisone 5 mg
    #20 is $1.73?

4. What is the co-pay for a prescription of Flagyl 250 mg #30 if the plan
    requires generic substitution and the co-pay is 20% of the usual and
    customary price? The usual and customary price for metronidazole
    250 mg #30 is $12.08 and the usual and customary price for Flagyl
    250 mg #30 is $34.77?

5. What is the co-pay for a prescription of Aldactone 25 mg #30 if the co-pay is $5 for generic and $10 for brand names and the usual and customary price for spironolactone 25 mg #30 is $12.08?

Calculate the difference price if the difference price is the sum of the co-pay amount + the difference in cost of the brand and generic.

6. What is the co-pay for a prescription of brand name Vicodin 5/500 #30 if there is no DAW on the prescription, but the patient wants to pay the difference pricing for the brand name? The co-pay amount is $5, the cost of Vicodin #30 is $18.05, and the cost of the generic #30 is $5.05.

7. What is the co-pay for a prescription of brand name Tenormin 50 mg #30 if there is no DAW on the prescription, but the patient wants to pay the difference pricing for the brand name? The co-pay amount is $10, the cost of Tenomrin 50 mg #30 is $35.40, and the cost of the generic #30 is $5.40.

8. What is the co-pay for a prescription of brand name Zestril 5 mg #30 if there is no DAW on the prescription, but the patient wants to pay the difference pricing for the brand name? The co-pay amount is $15, the cost of Zestril 5 mg #30 is $26.40, and the cost of the generic #30 is $15.40

9. What is the co-pay for a prescription of brand name Xanax 0.5 mg #30 if there is no DAW on the prescription, but the patient wants to pay the difference pricing for the brand name? The co-pay amount is $5, the cost of Xanax 0.5 mg #30 is $26.40, and the cost of the generic #30 is $3.40.

10.   What is the co-pay for a prescription of brand name Keflex 500 mg #30 if there is no DAW on the prescription, but the patient wants to pay the difference pricing for the brand name? The co-pay amount is $15, the cost of Keflex 500 mg #30 is $84.40, and the cost of the generic is $2.40.

11.   What is the co-pay for a prescription for brand name Glucophage 500 mg #60 if there is no DAW on the prescription, but the patient wants to pay the difference pricing for the brand name? The co-pay amount is $20, the cost of Glucophage 500 mg #60 is $39.60, and the cost of the generic is $28.40.

12.   What is the co-pay for a prescription for brand name Prozac 20 mg #30 if there is no DAW on the prescription, but the patient wants to pay the difference pricing for the brand name? The co-pay amount is $15, the cost of Prozac 20 mg #30 is $85.40, and the cost of the generic is $25.70.

13.   What is the co-pay for a prescription for brand name Ativan 1 mg #30 if there is no DAW on the prescription, but the patient wants to pay the difference pricing for the brand name? The co-pay amount is $15, the cost of Ativan 1 mg #30 is $32.10, and the cost of the generic is $6.80.

14.   What is the co-pay for a prescription for brand name Augmentin 500 mg #30 if there is no DAW on the prescription, but the patient wants to pay the difference pricing for the brand name? The co-pay amount is $20, the cost of Augmentin 500 mg #30 is $108.20, and the cost of the generic is $88.10.

15.   What is the co-pay for a prescription for brand name Klonopin 1 mg #30 if there is no DAW on the prescription, but the patient wants to pay the difference pricing for the brand name. The co-pay amount is $15, the cost of Klonopin 1 mg #30 is $26.40, and the cost of the generic is $6.40.

16.   What is the co-pay for a prescription for brand name Bactrim DS #20 if there is no DAW on the prescription, but the patient wants to pay the difference pricing for the brand name. The co-pay amount is $20, the cost of Bactrim DS #20 is $38.40, and the cost of the generic is $3.90.

17.   What is the co-pay for a prescription for brand name Desyrel 100 mg #30 if there is no DAW on the prescription, but the patient wants to pay the difference pricing for the brand name. The co-pay amount is $25, the cost of Desyrel 100 mg #30 is $88.60, and the cost of the generic is $4.90.

18.   What is the co-pay for a prescription for brand name Flexeril 10 mg #30 if there is no DAW on the prescription, but the patient wants to pay the difference pricing for the brand name. The co-pay amount is $20, the cost of Flexeril 10 mg #30 is $28.40, and the cost of the generic is $3.90.

19.   What is the co-pay for a prescription for Vasotec 10 mg #30 if there is no DAW on the prescription, but the patient wants to pay the difference pricing for the brand name. The co-pay amount is $15, the cost of Vasotec 10 mg #30 is $28.10, and the cost of the generic is $5.20.

20.   What is the co-pay for a prescription for Valium 10 mg #30 if there is no DAW on the prescription, but the patient wants to pay the difference pricing for the brand name. The co-pay amount is $12, the cost of Valium 10 mg #30 is $63.20, and the cost of the generic is $5.30.

21.   What is the co-pay for a prescription for Ultram 50 mg #30 if there is no DAW on the prescription, but the patient wants to pay the difference pricing for the brand name. The co-pay amount is $20, the cost of Ultram 50 mg #30 is $22.80, and the cost of the generic is $10.40.

22.   What is the co-pay for a prescription for Soma 350 mg #30 if there is no DAW on the prescription, but the patient wants to pay the difference pricing for the brand name. The co-pay amount is $15, the cost of Soma 350 mg #30 is $108.10, and the cost of the generic is $5.40.

23.   What is the co-pay for a prescription for Calan SR 240 mg #30 if there is no DAW on the prescription, but the patient wants to pay the difference pricing for the brand name. The co-pay amount is $20, the cost of Calan SR 240 mg is $54.20, and the cost of the generic is $5.90.

24.   What is the co-pay for a prescription for Vibramycin 100 mg #20 if there is no DAW on the prescription, but the patient wants to pay the difference pricing for the brand name. The co-pay amount is $15, the cost of Vibramycin 100 mg #20 is $91.40, and the cost of the generic is $4.90.

25. What is the co-pay for a prescription for Imdur 30 mg #30 if there is no DAW on the prescription, but the patient wants to pay the difference pricing for the brand name. The co-pay amount is $20, the cost of Imdur 30 mg #30 is $42.80, and the cost of the generic is $9.20.

20 Calculations for Billing Compounds

ALCULATIONS FOR BILLING COMPOUNDS are determined by a contractual agreement by the third party and the pharmacy. The formula that should be used can vary among different third parties. Often, the formula is determined by the cost of the ingredients + a dispensing fee + a fee for the time it took to prepare the compound.

Example:

How much should an insurance company be billed for the following compound if the compound was prepared in 20 minutes and the dispensing fee is $3.25?

Hydrocortisone 2.5% in Eucerin Cream
Dispense 60 gm
Sig: Apply sparingly b.i.d. prn

1. Calculate how much hydrocortisone is needed:

   2.5 gm HC/100 gm total × 60 gm total = 1.5 gm HC

2. Calculate the cost of the hydrocortisone (hydrocortisone comes in a 10 gm container that costs the pharmacy $31.25).

   1.5 gm HC × $31.25/10 gm HC = $4.69

3. Calculate how much Eucerin cream is needed:

   Total weight = weight of hydrocortisone + weight of Eucerin cream

   Using algebra, you can solve for the weight of the Eucerin cream

   Weight of Eucerin cream = total weight − weight of hydrocortisone

   Weight of Eucerin cream = 60 gm − 1.5 gm = 58.5 gm

4. Calculate the cost of the Eucerin if Eucerin comes from a 454 gm jar that costs the pharmacy $15.45:

   58.5 gm × $15.45/454 gm = $1.99

5. The amount to be billed is determined by adding the cost of the ingredients + the dispensing fee + the cost of the time to prepare the compound. You must next determine the cost of time to prepare the prescription:

20 min × 1 hr/60 min × $35.00/hr = $11.67

So the total amount of the prescription is:

$3.25	+	$4.69	+	$1.99	+	$11.67	=	$21.60
dispensing fee		cost of HC		cost of Eucerin		cost of time		total

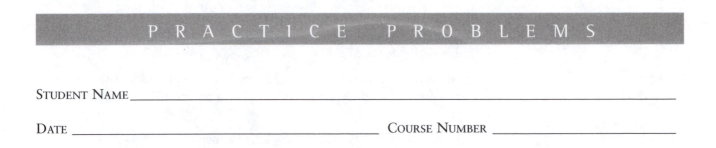

P R A C T I C E   P R O B L E M S

STUDENT NAME _____

DATE _____ COURSE NUMBER _____

For the following problems use $35.00/hr to calculate the cost of time to prepare the prescription.

1. How much should an insurance company be billed for the following compound if the compound was prepared in 30 minutes and the dispensing fee is $3.25?

   Ibuprofen 10% cream 30 grams
   Cost of ingredients = $12.47

2. How much should an insurance company be billed for the following compound if the compound was prepared in 10 minutes and the dispensing fee is $3.25?

   Clindamycin phosphate 600 mg in Cetaphil Lotion
   Dispense 60 ml
   Sig: Apply hs ud

   Costs:
   Clindamycin phosphate 600 mg/ampule = $6.19
   Cetaphil Lotion 240 ml = $9.49

3. How much should an insurance company be billed for the following compound if the compound was prepared in 20 minutes and the dispensing fee is $3.25?

   Hydrocortisone 2.5% in Eucerin Cream
   Dispense 60 gm
   Sig: Apply sparingly b.i.d. prn

   Costs:
   Hydrocortisone Powder 10 gm = $53.80
   Eucerin Cream 400 gm = $8.27

4. How much should an insurance company be billed for the following compound if the compound was prepared in 20 minutes and the dispensing fee is $3.25?

    Tetracycline HCl suspension 125 mg/5 ml compounded from capsules and a mixture of Ora-Plus 50% and Ora-Sweet 50% q.s. 200 ml

    Costs:
    Tetracycline 250 mg capsules = $0.23/capsule
    Ora-Plus 473 ml = $9.47
    Ora-Sweet 473 ml = $9.47

5. How much should an insurance company be billed for the following compound if the compound was prepared in 20 minutes and the dispensing fee is $3.25?

    Metoprolol tartrate 10 mg/ml Oral Liquid in a 50:50 mixture of Ora-Sweet:Ora Plus Vehicle q.s. 120 ml

    Costs:
    Metoprolol tartrate 100 mg = $0.35/tablet
    Ora-Plus 473 ml = $9.47
    Ora-Sweet 473 ml = $9.47

6. How much should be charged for salicylic acid 1%, menthol 1/4% in triamcinolone 0.1% cream 60 gm if the dispensing fee is $4.25, the cost of ingredients is $8.40, and the compound was prepared in 20 minutes?

7. How much should be charged for menthol 1/4% in triamcinolone 0.1% cream 30 gm if the dispensing fee is $4.25, the cost of ingredients is $4.40, and the compound was prepared in 20 minutes?

8. How much should be charged for 170 ml diphenhydramine elixir, 50 ml lidocaine viscous, 200 ml nystatin suspension, 52 ml of erythromycin ethyl succinate suspension, and 28 ml of cherry syrup to make 500 ml if the dispensing fee is $4.25, the cost of ingredients is $18.40, and the compound was prepared in 20 minutes?

9. How much should be charged for 100 ml of hydrocortisone 2 mg/ml if the dispensing fee is $4.25, the cost of ingredients is $22.20, and the compound was prepared in 18 minutes?

10. How much should be charged for 70 ml of lansoprazole 3 mg/ml suspension if the dispensing fee is $4.25, the cost of ingredients is $38.14, and the compound was prepared in 15 minutes?

11. How much should be charged for 120 ml of potassium bromide 250 mg/ml if the dispensing fee is $4.25, the cost of ingredients is $6.25, and the compound was prepared in 10 minutes?

12. How much should be charged for 150 ml of clonidine 0.1 mg/5 ml suspension if the dispensing fee is $4.25, the cost of ingredients is $5.30, and the compound was prepared in 20 minutes?

13.   How much should be charged for 300 ml of methylphenidate 10 mg/5 ml suspension if the dispensing fee is $4.25, the cost of ingredients is $36.20, and the compound was prepared in 15 minutes?

14.   How much should be charged for 50 ml of captopril 1 mg/ml suspension if the dispensing fee is $4.25, the cost of ingredients is $0.85, and the compound was prepared in 20 minutes?

15.   How much should be charged for 45 ml of baclofen 10 mg/ml if the dispensing fee is $4.25, the cost of ingredients is $7.25, and the compound was prepared in 20 minutes?

16.   How much should be charged for 15 ml of amiptriptyline 20 mg/ml suspension if the dispensing fee is $4.25, the cost of ingredients is $8.70, and the compound was prepared in 15 minutes?

17.   How much should be charged for 90 ml of hydrochlorothiazide 10 mg/ml if the dispensing fee is $4.25, the cost of ingredients is $4.20, and the compound was prepared in 15 minutes?

18. How much should be charged for 30 gm of salicylic acid 40% in petrolatum if the dispensing fee is $4.25, the cost of ingredients is $11.40, and the compound was prepared in 20 minutes?

19. How much should be charged for 150 ml of metformin 100 mg/ml suspension if the dispensing fee is $4.25, the cost of ingredients is $38.10, and the compound was prepared in 20 minutes?

20. How much should be charged for 150 ml of metronidazole 59 mg/5 ml suspension if the dispensing fee is $4.25, the cost of ingredients is $16.20, and the compound was prepared in 20 minutes?

21. How much should be charged for 60 ml of enalapril 1 mg/ml suspension if the dispensing fee is $4.25, the cost of ingredients is $19.10, and the compound was prepared in 20 minutes?

22. How much should be charged for 120 ml of amiodarone 5 mg/ml suspension if the dispensing fee is $4.25, the cost of ingredients is $22.70, and the compound was prepared in 20 minutes?

23.   How much should be charged for hydrocortisone 2.4 g in 240 ml
Lubriderm lotion if the dispensing fee is $4.25, the cost of ingredients
is $21.50, and the compound was prepared in 20 minutes?

24.   How much should be charged for 100 ml of celecoxib 100 mg/5 ml if
the dispensing fee is $4.25, the cost of ingredients is $21.15, and the
compound was prepared in 15 minutes?

25.   How much should be charged for 240 ml PAC syrup if the dispensing
fee is $4.25, the cost of ingredients is $32.20, and the compound was
prepared in 20 minutes?

21 Cash Register Calculations

MOST CASH REGISTERS IN USE TODAY automatically calculate how much change is due when a customer pays. However, some cash registers do not automatically make this calculation, and sometimes patients or customers pay with a different amount of money than the amount entered into the cash register. Therefore, it is helpful to know how to do these calculations.

Example:

The price of a prescription is $15.45 and the patient pays with $20. How much change should you give to the patient?

To solve this problem, the change can be counted back to the patient in the following way:

1. 1 nickel makes $15.50

2. 2 quarters makes $16.00

3. 4 one dollar bills makes $20.00

The patient/customer is given $4.55.

Example:

The price of a prescription is $6.23 and the patient pays with $50. How much change is due in pennies, nickels, dimes, quarters, dollar bills, five dollar bills, ten dollar bills, and twenty dollar bills?

To solve the problem, the change can be counted back to the patient in the following way:

1. 2 pennies makes $6.25

2. 3 quarters makes $7.00

3. 3 one dollar bills makes $10.00

4. 2 twenty dollar bills makes $50.00

The patient/customer is given $43.77

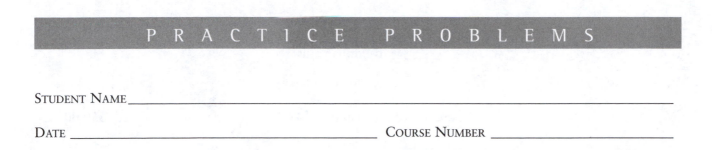

PRACTICE PROBLEMS

STUDENT NAME_____

DATE _____ COURSE NUMBER _____

Calculate the amount of change due in pennies, nickels, dimes, quarters, dollar bills, five dollar bills, ten dollar bills, and twenty dollar bills for the following transactions:

1. Amount of prescription: $16.41   Amount tendered: $50.00

    _____ pennies

    _____ nickels

    _____ dimes

    _____ quarters

    _____ one dollar bills

    _____ five dollar bills

    _____ ten dollar bills

    _____ twenty dollar bills

2. Amount of prescription: $35.22   Amount tendered: $50.00

    _____ pennies

    _____ nickels

    _____ dimes

    _____ quarters

    _____ one dollar bills

    _____ five dollar bills

    _____ ten dollar bills

3. Amount of prescription: $6.12   Amount tendered: $20.00

    _____ pennies

    _____ nickels

    _____ dimes

    _____ quarters

_____ one dollar bills

_____ five dollar bills

_____ ten dollar bills

4.   Amount of prescription: $42.50   Amount tendered: $50.00

_____ pennies

_____ nickels

_____ dimes

_____ quarters

_____ one dollar bills

_____ five dollar bills

5.   Amount of prescription: $22.22   Amount tendered: $30.00

_____ pennies

_____ nickels

_____ dimes

_____ quarters

_____ one dollar bills

_____ five dollar bills

6.   Amount of prescription: $26.25   Amount tendered: $40.00

_____ pennies

_____ nickels

_____ dimes

_____ quarters

_____ one dollar bills

_____ five dollar bills

_____ ten dollar bills

7.   Amount of prescription: $1.03   Amount tendered: $50.00

_____ pennies

_____ nickels

_____ dimes

_____ quarters

_____ one dollar bills

_____ five dollar bills

_____ ten dollar bills

_____ twenty dollar bills

8. Amount of prescription: $44.41   Amount tendered: $60.00

_____ pennies

_____ nickels

_____ dimes

_____ quarters

_____ one dollar bills

_____ five dollar bills

_____ ten dollar bills

9. Amount of prescription: $9.80   Amount tendered: $100.00

_____ pennies

_____ nickels

_____ dimes

_____ quarters

_____ one dollar bills

_____ five dollar bills

_____ ten dollar bills

_____ twenty dollar bills

10. Amount of prescription: $12.06   Amount tendered: $50.06

_____ pennies

_____ nickels

_____ dimes

_____ quarters

_____ one dollar bills

_____ five dollar bills

_____ ten dollar bills

_____ twenty dollar bills

11.   Amount of prescription: $63.12   Amount tendered: $70.00

_____ pennies

_____ nickels

_____ dimes

_____ quarters

_____ one dollar bills

_____ five dollar bills

_____ ten dollar bills

_____ twenty dollar bills

12.   Amount of prescription: $41.59   Amount tendered: $50.00

_____ pennies

_____ nickels

_____ dimes

_____ quarters

_____ one dollar bills

_____ five dollar bills

_____ ten dollar bills

_____ twenty dollar bills

13.   Amount of prescription: $163.12   Amount tendered: $180.00

_____ pennies

_____ nickels

_____ dimes

_____ quarters

_____ one dollar bills

_____ five dollar bills

_____ ten dollar bills

_____ twenty dollar bills

14. Amount of prescription: $23.55   Amount tendered: $40.00

_____ pennies

_____ nickels

_____ dimes

_____ quarters

_____ one dollar bills

_____ five dollar bills

_____ ten dollar bills

_____ twenty dollar bills

15. Amount of prescription: $89.04   Amount tendered: $100.04

_____ pennies

_____ nickels

_____ dimes

_____ quarters

_____ one dollar bills

_____ five dollar bills

_____ ten dollar bills

_____ twenty dollar bills

16. Amount of prescription: $113.42   Amount tendered: $200.00

_____ pennies

_____ nickels

_____ dimes

_____ quarters

_____ one dollar bills

_____ five dollar bills

_____ ten dollar bills

_____ twenty dollar bills

17.   Amount of prescription: $3.82   Amount tendered: $20.00

_____ pennies

_____ nickels

_____ dimes

_____ quarters

_____ one dollar bills

_____ five dollar bills

_____ ten dollar bills

_____ twenty dollar bills

18.   Amount of prescription: $18.99   Amount tendered: $50.00

_____ pennies

_____ nickels

_____ dimes

_____ quarters

_____ one dollar bills

_____ five dollar bills

_____ ten dollar bills

_____ twenty dollar bills

19.   Amount of prescription: $198.89   Amount tendered: $200.00

_____ pennies

_____ nickels

_____ dimes

_____ quarters

_____ one dollar bills

_____ five dollar bills

_____ ten dollar bills

_____ twenty dollar bills

20.   Amount of prescription: $311.44   Amount tendered: $320.00

_____ pennies

_____ nickels

_____ dimes

_____ quarters

_____ one dollar bills

_____ five dollar bills

_____ ten dollar bills

_____ twenty dollar bills

21.   Amount of prescription: $5.05   Amount tendered: $20.05

_____ pennies

_____ nickels

_____ dimes

_____ quarters

_____ one dollar bills

_____ five dollar bills

_____ ten dollar bills

_____ twenty dollar bills

22.   Amount of prescription: $59.98   Amount tendered: $60.03

_____ pennies

_____ nickels

_____ dimes

_____ quarters

_____ one dollar bills

_____ five dollar bills

_____ ten dollar bills

_____ twenty dollar bills

23.   Amount of prescription: $115.52   Amount tendered: $120.02

_____ pennies

_____ nickels

_____ dimes

_____ quarters

_____ one dollar bills

_____ five dollar bills

_____ ten dollar bills

_____ twenty dollar bills

24.   Amount of prescription: $10.98   Amount tendered: $20.00

_____ pennies

_____ nickels

_____ dimes

_____ quarters

_____ one dollar bills

_____ five dollar bills

_____ ten dollar bills

_____ twenty dollar bills

25.   Amount of prescription: $71.51   Amount tendered: $80.01

_____ pennies

_____ nickels

_____ dimes

_____ quarters

_____ one dollar bills

_____ five dollar bills

_____ ten dollar bills

_____ twenty dollar bills

26. Amount of prescription: $49.53   Amount tendered: $50.03

_____ pennies

_____ nickels

_____ dimes

_____ quarters

_____ one dollar bills

_____ five dollar bills

_____ ten dollar bills

_____ twenty dollar bills

27. Amount of prescription: $101.37   Amount tendered: $120.00

_____ pennies

_____ nickels

_____ dimes

_____ quarters

_____ one dollar bills

_____ five dollar bills

_____ ten dollar bills

_____ twenty dollar bills

28. Amount of prescription: $57.84   Amount tendered: $60.00

_____ pennies

_____ nickels

_____ dimes

_____ quarters

_____ one dollar bills

_____ five dollar bills

_____ ten dollar bills

_____ twenty dollar bills

29.   Amount of prescription: $143.32   Amount tendered: $160.00

_____ pennies

_____ nickels

_____ dimes

_____ quarters

_____ one dollar bills

_____ five dollar bills

_____ ten dollar bills

_____ twenty dollar bills

30.   Amount of prescription: $48.45   Amount tendered: $100.00

_____ pennies

_____ nickels

_____ dimes

_____ quarters

_____ one dollar bills

_____ five dollar bills

_____ ten dollar bills

_____ twenty dollar bills

22 Usual and Customary Prices

THE USUAL AND CUSTOMARY PRICE (U&C) is the price charged to patients who pay cash for prescriptions. U&C prices are usually determined in the corporate offices. For some new medications and medications that are rarely used, U&C prices are sometimes determined in the pharmacy using a formula provided by corporate management. This formula may already be programmed into the pharmacy computer system so the U&C price can be determined automatically when a prescription is filled.

Example:

If prescription prices are determined using the following formula:

AWP + professional fee = selling price of prescription

The professional fee is determined using the following chart:

AWP	Professional Fee
Less than $20.00	$4.00
$20.01 – $50.00	$5.00
Greater than $50.01	$6.00

Example:

If the AWP for 30 capsules of amoxicillin 250 mg is $3.50, what will be the selling price of the prescription?

Since the AWP for the prescription is less than $20.00, the professional fee is $4.00.

Using the formula:

AWP + professional fee = selling price of prescription

$3.50 + $4.00 = $7.50

Some pharmacies sell certain medications at a price lower than the acquisition cost. Therefore, the usual and customary price may be less than the average wholesale price (AWP) or less than the acquisition cost. Many third-party plans reimburse the pharmacy based on the lowest amount: AWP, acquisition cost, or U&C, since the third parties do not want to pay more for a prescription than the patient would pay in cash.

Example:

A prescription is filled for one 10 ml bottle of NPH U-100 insulin. The AWP for one 10 ml bottle of NPH U-100 is $17.45. The acquisition cost to the pharmacy is $16.70. The usual and customary price for one bottle of NPH U-100 insulin at that pharmacy is $14.99.

If the pharmacy has an agreement with the third-party plan for reimbursement of 87% AWP or 100% U&C (whichever is less) + a $3.50 dispensing fee, what will be the total amount of the third-party claim?

First, determine the lowest cost basis for calculation of the third-party claim.

$.87 \times \$17.45 = \$15.18$

$15.18 (87% AWP) is greater than $14.99 (U&C), therefore calculation of the third-party claim will be based on the lower amount.

The total third-party claim will be $14.99 + $3.50 = $18.49.

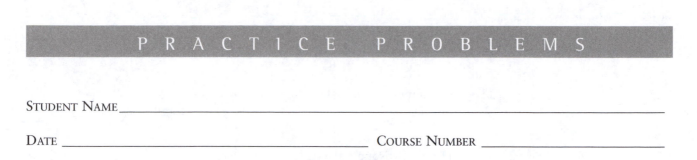

STUDENT NAME _____

DATE _____   COURSE NUMBER _____

Calculate the retail price of the following prescriptions using the formula AWP + professional fee = retail price of prescription if the professional fee is determined using the following chart:

AWP	Professional Fee
less than $20.00	$4.00
$20.01 – $50.00	$5.00
Greater than $50.01	$6.00

1. Verapamil SR Tabs #30 AWP/100 $120.85   retail price _____

2. Glyburide 5 mg Tabs #30 AWP/1000 $440.05   retail price _____

3. Dexamethasone 4 mg Tabs #12 AWP/100 $58.40   retail price _____

4. Danazol 200 mg Caps #100 AWP/100 $306.38   retail price _____

5. Doxepin 150 mg Caps #30 AWP/100 $66.50   retail price _____

6. Tetracycline 250 mg Caps #28 AWP/1000 $52.43   retail price _____

7. Docusate Calcium 240 mg Caps #30 AWP/100 $9.90   retail price _____

8. Amantadine Syrup 4 oz. AWP/PINT $61.51   retail price _____

9. Fluocinolone Cream 0.025% 15 Gm AWP/15 GM $3.05   retail price _____

10.   Acebutolol 400 mg Caps #60
        AWP/100 $121.51   retail price _____

11.   Guanabenz 4 mg Tabs #30 AWP/100
        $66.20   retail price _____

12.   Hydrocortisone Valerate Cream 0.2%
        45 GM AWP/45 GM $28.14   retail price _____

13.   Hydrocodone/APAP 5/500 #30
        AWP/100 $14.80   retail price _____

14.   Atenolol 50 mg #30 AWP/100
        $5.20   retail price _____

15.   Amoxicillin 250 mg #30 AWP/100
        $2.20   retail price _____

16.   Lisinopril 10 mg #30 AWP/100
        $14.40   retail price _____

17.   Hydrochlorothiazide 25 mg #30
        AWP/100 $4.80   retail price _____

18.   Furosemide Oral 20 mg #30 AWP/100
        $5.40   retail price _____

19.   Albuterol Aerosol 17 gm AWP/17 gm
        $8.40   retail price _____

20.   Alprazolam 0.25 mg #30 AWP/100
        $5.60   retail price _____

21.   Cephalexin 500 mg #40 AWP/100
        $19.60   retail price _____

22.   Triamterene w/HCTZ 37.5 mg/25 mg
        AWP/100 $12.10   retail price _____

If the pharmacy has an agreement with the third party plan for reimbursement of 87% AWP or 100% U&C (whichever is less) + a $3.50 dispensing fee, what will be the total amount of the third party claim for the following prescriptions?

23. Verapamil Sr Tabs #30 AWP/100
    $120.85 retail price/30 $40.20   amount of claim_____

24. Danazol 200 mg Caps #100 AWP/100
    $306.38 retail price/30 $95.39   amount of claim_____

25. Doxepin 150 mg Caps #30 AWP/100
    $66.50 retail price/30 $28.60   amount of claim_____

26. Tetracycline 250 mg Caps #28
    AWP/1000 $52.43 retail price/28 $6.99   amount of claim_____

27. Amantadine Syrup 4 oz. AWP/PINT
    $61.51 retail price/4 oz. $28.60   amount of claim_____

28. Amitriptyline 50 mg #90 AWP/100
    $5.40 retail price/90 $8.99   amount of claim_____

29. Clonazepam 1 mg #30 AWP/100
    $15.20 retail price/90 $22.59   amount of claim_____

30. Warfarin 5 mg #30 AWP/100 $29.90
    retail price/30 $15.99   amount of claim_____

31. Trimethoprim/Sulfa #20 AWP/100
    $12.30 retail price/30 $8.99   amount of claim_____

32. Trazodone 50 mg #30 AWP/100
    $11.40 retail price/30 $8.99   amount of claim_____

33. Cyclobenzaprine 10 mg #30 AWP/100
    $14.30 retail price/30 $8.49   amount of claim_____

34.   Enalapril 20 mg #30 AWP/100 $13.90
        retail price/30 $11.99   amount of claim_____

35.   Carisoprodol 350 mg #30 AWP/100
        $24.80 retail price/30 $17.99   amount of claim_____

36.   Verapamil SR 180 mg #30 AWP/100
        $15.60 retail price/30 $12.99   amount of claim_____

37.   Doxycycline 100 mg #20 AWP/100
        $33.40 retail price/20 $12.99   amount of claim_____

23 Discounts

PHARMACIES SOMETIMES GIVE a 5% or 10% discount on the price of prescriptions to certain patients such as senior citizens who are not participating in third party programs. State pharmacy regulations or third party contractual agreements may prohibit discounting prescriptions that are covered by third party programs. Sometimes, the discount is restricted to prescriptions purchased on certain days of the week.

Example:

A senior citizen is paying for a prescription for amoxicillin 250 mg #30. The usual and customary price is $8.49; however this patient qualifies for a 10% discount. How much will the patient pay?

$8.49 – 10\% (\$8.49) = \$8.49 – (0.1)(\$8.49) = \$8.49 – \$0.85 = \$7.64$

STUDENT NAME_____

DATE _____ COURSE NUMBER _____

Calculate how much the patient will pay for the following prescriptions if the patient qualifies for a 5% discount:

1. Retail price for
    prescription is $4.99   after 5% discount the patient pays _____

2. Retail price for
    prescription is $12.47   after 5% discount the patient pays _____

3. Retail price for
    prescription is $35.20   after 5% discount the patient pays _____

4. Retail price for
    prescription is $89.90   after 5% discount the patient pays _____

5. Retail price for
    prescription is
    $120.47   after 5% discount the patient pays _____

6. Retail prices for
    prescriptions are
    $5.60 + $27.50   after 5% discount the patient pays _____

7. Retail prices for
    prescriptions are
    $22.10 + $68.50   after 5% discount the patient pays _____

8. Retail prices for
    prescriptions are
    $21.60 + $153.50   after 5% discount the patient pays _____

9. Retail prices for
    prescriptions are
    $5.60 + $67.12   after 5% discount the patient pays _____

10. Retail prices for
    prescriptions are
    $97.60 + $127.30   after 5% discount the patient pays _____

11. Retail price for prescriptions are $5.40 + $9.90 + $15.20   after 5% discount the patient pays _____

12. Retail price for prescriptions are $15.20 + $8.30 + $95.20   after 5% discount the patient pays _____

13. Retail price for prescriptions are $42.15 + $18.25 + $195.20   after 5% discount the patient pays _____

14. Retail price for prescriptions are $65.20 + $78.20 + $19.10   after 5% discount the patient pays _____

15. Retail price for prescriptions are $95.45 + $18.30 + $75.20   after 5% discount the patient pays _____

16. Retail price for prescriptions are $121.20 + $118.30 + $135.20   after 5% discount the patient pays _____

17. Retail price for prescriptions are $83.19 + $118.23 + $45.79   after 5% discount the patient pays _____

18. Retail price for prescriptions are $111.11 + $88.30 + $35.27   after 5% discount the patient pays _____

19. Retail price for prescriptions are $66.30 + $118.15 + $125.20   after 5% discount the patient pays _____

20. Retail price for prescriptions are $118.20 + $183.20 + $192.50   after 5% discount the patient pays _____

Calculate how much the patient will pay for the following prescriptions if the patient qualifies for a 10% discount:

21. Retail price for prescription is $4.99   after 10% discount the patient pays _____

22. Retail price for prescription is $12.47   after 10% discount the patient pays _____

23. Retail price for prescription is $35.20   after 10% discount the patient pays _____

24. Retail price for prescription is $89.90   after 10% discount the patient pays _____

25. Retail price for prescription is $120.47   after 10% discount the patient pays _____

26. Retail prices for prescriptions are $5.60 + $27.50   after 10% discount the patient pays _____

27. Retail prices for prescriptions are $22.10 + $68.50   after 10% discount the patient pays _____

28. Retail prices for prescriptions are $21.60 + $153.50   after 10% discount the patient pays _____

29. Retail prices for prescriptions are $5.60 + $67.12   after 10% discount the patient pays _____

30. Retail prices for prescriptions are $97.60 + $127.30   after 10% discount the patient pays _____

31. Retail price for prescriptions are $123.52 + $118.33 + $95.27   after 10% discount the patient pays _____

32.   Retail price for
prescriptions are
$15.29 +
$118.30 +
$9.20   after 10% discount the patient pays _____

33.   Retail price for
prescriptions are
$135.20 +
$82.30 +
$135.30   after 10% discount the patient pays _____

34.   Retail price for
prescriptions are
$125.24 +
$18.23 +
$93.23   after 10% discount the patient pays _____

35.   Retail price for
prescriptions are
$15.32 + $8.35 +
$65.29   after 10% discount the patient pays _____

36.   Retail price for
prescriptions are
$115.30 +
$18.40 +
$15.32   after 10% discount the patient pays _____

37.   Retail price for
prescriptions are
$125.10 +
$18.70 +
$90.10   after 10% discount the patient pays _____

38.   Retail price for
prescriptions are
$19.90 + $18.80 +
$15.50   after 10% discount the patient pays _____

39.   Retail price for
prescriptions are
$15.66 +
$112.30 +
$155.23   after 10% discount the patient pays _____

40.   Retail price for
prescriptions are
$15.55 + $8.88 +
$95.60   after 10% discount the patient pays _____

24 Gross and Net Profits

GROSS PROFIT IS THE DIFFERENCE between the selling price and acquisition price of an item, while net profit is the difference between the selling price and all associated costs (including the acquisition price).

Gross Profit

The gross profit is the difference between the selling price and the acquisition cost. For cash prescriptions, the selling price is the usual and customary price for prescriptions paid by cash customers. For third party prescriptions, the selling price is determined by a contractual agreement for prescriptions paid by third parties. To calculate gross profit, there is no consideration for any of the expenses associated with filling the prescription.

Gross profit = selling price − acquisition cost

The gross profit can be expressed as a percent.

Example:

A prescription for amoxicillin 250 mg #30 has a usual and customary price of $8.49. The acquisition cost of amoxicillin 250 mg #30 is $2.02. What is the gross profit?

Gross profit = selling price − acquisition cost

Gross profit = $8.49 − $2.02 = $6.47

Net Profit

The net profit is the difference between the selling price of the prescription and the sum of all the costs associated with filling the prescription. All the costs associated with filling the prescription include the cost of the medication, the cost of the container, the cost of the label, the cost of the bag, the cost of the labor to dispense the prescription, a portion of the rent, etc. For practical purposes, all the other costs can be grouped together and considered as a dispensing fee. Since the costs associated with operation of a pharmacy vary, the dispensing fee can vary.

Net profit = selling price − acquisition cost − dispensing fee

or

Net profit = gross profit − dispensing fee

Net profit can also be expressed as a percent.

Example:

A prescription for amoxicillin 250 mg #30 has a usual and customary price of $8.49. The acquisition cost of amoxicillin 250 mg #30 is $2.02. What is the net profit if the dispensing fee/professional fee is $5.50?

Net profit = selling price − acquisition cost − dispensing fee

Net profit = $8.49 − $2.02 − $5.50 = $0.97

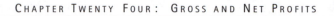

PRACTICE PROBLEMS

STUDENT NAME_____

DATE _____ COURSE NUMBER _____

Use this table to determine the dispensing/professional fee:

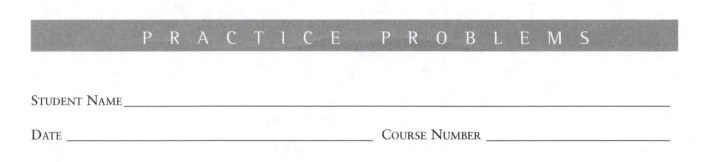

AWP	Dispensing/Professional Fee
less than $20.00	$4.00
$20.01 – $50.00	$5.00
Greater than $50.01	$6.00

then calculate the gross profit and the net profit for the following prescriptions:

1. Zocor 5 mg, 60 tablets, acquisition cost = $85.47, AWP = $106.84, selling price = $109.93

   Gross profit = _____   Net profit = _____

2. Prilosec 20 mg, 30 cap., acquisition cost = $99.20, AWP = $108.90, selling price = $116.38

   Gross profit = _____   Net profit = _____

3. Norvasc 5 mg, 90 tablets, acquisition cost = $97.92, WP = $125.66, selling price = $117.82

   Gross profit = _____   Net profit = _____

4. Procardia XL 30 mg, 100 tablets, acquisition cost = $105.05 AWP = $131.31, selling price = $134.36

   Gross profit = _____   Net profit = _____

5. Vasotec 10 mg, 100 tablets, acquisition cost = $85.56, AWP = $102.94, selling price = $109.19

   Gross profit = _____   Net profit = _____

6. Relafen 500 mg, 100 tablets, acquisition cost = $88.88, AWP = $111.10, selling price = $120.27

   Gross profit = _____   Net profit = _____

7. Zoloft 50 mg, 100 tablets, acquisition cost = $172.44, AWP = $215.55, selling price = $226.50

   Gross profit = _____   Net profit = _____

8. Fosamax 10 mg, 30 tablets, acquisition cost = $50.91,
   AWP = $51.88, selling price = $57.62

   Gross profit = _____   Net profit = _____

9. Cardizem CD 240 mg, 90 tablets, acquisition cost = $154.10,
   AWP = $165.42, selling price = $179.69

   Gross profit = _____   Net profit = _____

10. Ticlid 250 mg, 60 tablets, acquisition cost = $99.44,
    AWP = $108.90, selling price = $122.07

    Gross profit = _____   Net profit =_____

11. Atenolol 50 mg, 90 tablets, acquisition cost = $5.80,
    AWP = $9.80, selling price = $15.99

    Gross profit = _____   Net profit = _____

12. Amoxicillin 500 mg 90 capsules, acquisition cost = $7.80,
    AWP = $12.80, selling price = $18.99

    Gross profit = _____   Net profit = _____

13. Lisinopril 20 mg 90 tablets, acquisition cost = $35.80,
    AWP = $42.80, selling price = $45.99

    Gross profit = _____   Net profit = _____

14. Hydrochlorothiazide 50 mg 90 tablets, acquisition
    cost = $1.80, AWP = $4.80, selling price = $10.99

    Gross profit = _____   Net profit = _____

15. Furosemide 20 mg 90 tablets, acquisition cost = $3.20,
    AWP = $7.90, selling price = $10.99

    Gross profit = _____   Net profit = _____

16. Albuterol Aerosol 17 gm, acquisition cost = $8.80,
    AWP = $11.80, selling price = $15.99

    Gross profit = _____   Net profit = _____

17. Alprazolam 1 mg 90 tablets, acquisition cost = $4.90,
    AWP = $9.80, selling price = $17.99

    Gross profit = _____   Net profit = _____

18. Prednisone 10 mg 90 tablets, acquisition cost = $2.80,
    AWP = $8.60, selling price = $12.99

    Gross profit = _____   Net profit = _____

19.   Metformin 500 mg 60 tablets, acquisition cost = $25.80,
AWP = $32.80, selling price = $36.99

Gross profit = _____   Net profit = _____

20.   Fluoxetine 20 mg 30 capsules, acquisition cost = $25.20,
AWP = $39.80, selling price = $45.99

Gross profit = _____   Net profit = _____

21.   Metoprolol 50 mg 60 tablets, acquisition cost = $5.20,
AWP = $8.80, selling price = $11.99

Gross profit = _____   Net profit = _____

22.   Lorazepam 1 mg 30 tablets, acquisition cost = $8.80,
AWP = $9.80, selling price = $15.99

Gross profit = _____   Net profit = _____

23.   Amitriptyline 25 mg 90 tablets, acquisition cost = $5.80,
AWP = $7.80, selling price = $12.99

Gross profit = _____   Net profit = _____

24.   Enalapril 5 mg 90 tablets, acquisition cost = $15.80,
AWP = $19.80, selling price = $25.99

Gross profit = _____   Net profit = _____

25.   Tramadol 50 mg 30 tablets, acquisition cost = $12.80,
AWP = $15.80, selling price = $22.99

Gross profit = _____   Net profit = _____

26.   Carisoprodol 350 mg 30 tablets, acquisition cost = $7.85,
AWP = $9.93, selling price = $15.99

Gross profit = _____   Net profit = _____

27.   Verapamil SR 120 mg 90 tablets, acquisition cost = $32.80,
AWP = $35.80, selling price = $45.99

Gross profit = _____   Net profit = _____

28.   Doxycycline 100 mg 20 capsules, acquisition cost = $5.20,
AWP = $6.70, selling price = $10.99

Gross profit = _____   Net profit = _____

29. Isosorbide Mononitrate 60 mg CR 30 tablets, acquisition
cost = $25.80, AWP = $29.90, selling price = $37.99

Gross profit = _____   Net profit = _____

30. Glyburide micronized 3 mg 60 tablets, acquisition
cost = $12.80, AWP = $19.80, selling price = $25.99

Gross profit = _____   Net profit = _____

25 Inventory Control

MOST PHARMACIES MUST BORROW MONEY and pay interest on the borrowed money in order to keep an adequate supply of medications on the shelf with which to fill all anticipated prescriptions. The amount paid toward the interest for borrowing money to keep drugs on the shelf affects the operating expenses and therefore affects the net profit or "bottom line."

Ideally, pharmacies could have all drugs on the shelf at all times; but this is practically impossible due to the high cost of medications. Although pharmacy technicians are usually not involved in securing loans for the pharmacy, they should have some appreciation for the expenses associated with maintaining an inventory and the significance of inventory control.

The expenses associated with borrowing money can be calculated using the following equation:

$$B = A (1 + r/n)^{NT} - P [(1 + r/n)^{NT} - 1]/[(1 + r/n) - 1]$$

where

> B = balance after t (or T) years
> A = amount borrowed
> n or N = number of payments per year
> P = amount paid per payment
> r = annual percentage rate (APR)

If an amount A is borrowed and will be repaid by n repayments per year, each of an amount P, interest will accumulate at an annual percentage rate of r, and this interest will compound n times a year (along with each payment). Installments will be of amount P until the original amount and any accumulated interest is repaid. This equation gives the amount B that will be repaid after t years.

Rather than working through this equation to calculate the expenses associated with borrowing money, computer programs or tables are usually used. Therefore, it is not practical for a pharmacy technician to solve problems using this equation, but it is important to have an appreciation for the expenses associated with maintaining an inventory of prescription drugs.

As the amount of money paid for interest on borrowed money increases, profits decrease. Therefore, in order to maximize profits, the pharmacy inventory should be as low as possible while having enough medication in stock to fill prescriptions.

Computerized methods for inventory control are evolving; however, human intervention is necessary for the computerized methods to be effective. Computerized methods can be based on minimum/maximum level inventory systems. In minimum/maximum level inventory systems, drugs are reordered up to the maximum inventory level when the minimum inventory level is reached.

The maximum inventory level – # bottle(s) on hand = order quantity (bottle(s))

Example:

Amoxicillin 250 mg capsules are stocked in 500 ct. bottles. The acquisition cost to the pharmacy for each 500 ct. bottle is $55.50. The shelf label indicates the minimum/maximum inventory level for amoxicillin 250 mg 500 ct. is 2/4. There is only a partial bottle on the shelf. Should this medication be reordered? If so, how many bottles should you order?

Answer: Since the minimum shelf quantity is 2 and there is only 1 bottle on the shelf, yes the medication should be reordered. The medication should be reordered up to the maximum shelf quantity.

The maximum inventory level – # bottle(s) on hand = order quantity (bottle(s))

4 bottles (maximum) – 1 bottle (on hand) = 3 bottles (order)

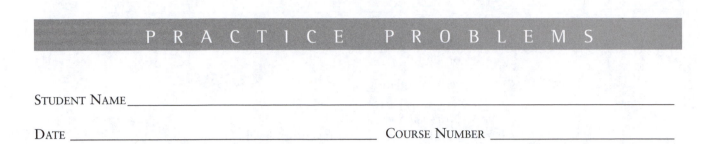

STUDENT NAME_____

DATE _____ COURSE NUMBER _____

Determine the reorder quantities for the following medication using information from the minimum/maximum inventory levels on the shelf labels and the on-hand quantities:

1. Ambien 5 mg
    minimum/maximum inventory level   1/2
    on hand   1

    reorder quantity   _____

2. Terazol-3
    minimum/maximum inventory level   6/12
    on hand   4

    reorder quantity   _____

3. Pepcid 20 mg
    minimum/maximum inventory level   2/5
    on hand   4

    reorder quantity   _____

4. Prozac 20 mg
    minimum/maximum inventory level   6/12
    on hand   1

    reorder quantity   _____

5. Nitrostat 0.4 mg 4 × 25s
    minimum/maximum inventory level   2/4
    on hand   3

    reorder quantity   _____

6. Tylenol #3 1000s
    minimum/maximum inventory level   1/2
    on hand   1

    reorder quantity   _____

7. Lipitor 10 mg
    minimum/maximum inventory level   3/10
    on hand   2

    reorder quantity   _____

8. Synthroid 0.05 mg
    minimum/maximum inventory level   2/4
    on hand   1

    reorder quantity   _____

9. Norvasc 5 mg
    minimum/maximum inventory level   3/7
    on hand   2

    reorder quantity   _____

10. Zoloft 50 mg
    minimum/maximum inventory level   3/5
    on hand   1

    reorder quantity   _____

11. Zithromax Z-Pak
    minimum/maximum inventory level   6/12
    on hand   5

    reorder quantity   _____

12. Toprol XL 50 mg
    minimum/maximum inventory level   1/2
    on hand   2

    reorder quantity   _____

13. Zocor 10 mg
    minimum/maximum inventory level   2/5
    on hand   2

    reorder quantity   _____

14. Prevacid 30 mg
    minimum/maximum inventory level   3/7
    on hand   3

    reorder quantity   _____

15. Premarin Tabs 0.625 mg
    minimum/maximum inventory level   1/2
    on hand   2

    reorder quantity   _____

16. Ambien 5 mg
    minimum/maximum inventory level   1/2
    on hand   2

    reorder quantity   _____

17.   Levoxyl 0.05 mg
      minimum/maximum inventory level   2/4
      on hand   4

      reorder quantity   _____

18.   Allegra 60 mg
      minimum/maximum inventory level   3/5
      on hand   3

      reorder quantity   _____

19.   Celebrex 200 mg
      minimum/maximum inventory level   2/4
      on hand   3

      reorder quantity   _____

20.   Nexium 40 mg
      minimum/maximum inventory level   3/10
      on hand   6

      reorder quantity   _____

21.   Zyrtec 10 mg
      minimum/maximum inventory level   2/3
      on hand   3

      reorder quantity   _____

22.   Singulair 10 mg
      minimum/maximum inventory level   3/5
      on hand   4

      reorder quantity   _____

23.   Vioxx 50 mg
      minimum/maximum inventory level   2/5
      on hand   3

      reorder quantity   _____

24.   Fosamax 10 mg
      minimum/maximum inventory level   2/4
      on hand   3

      reorder quantity   _____

25.   Effexor XR 75 mg
      minimum/maximum inventory level   3/7
      on hand   5

      reorder quantity   _____

26.   Neurontin 400 mg
        minimum/maximum inventory level   1/3
        on hand   2

        reorder quantity   _____

27.   Celexa 20 mg
        minimum/maximum inventory level   3/6
        on hand   6

        reorder quantity   _____

28.   Lexapro 20 mg
        minimum/maximum inventory level   2/4
        on hand   4

        reorder quantity   _____

26 Daily Cash Report

I N SOME RETAIL PHARMACY PRACTICES, pharmacy technicians assist the pharmacist with preparing the daily cash report for the entire store. Daily cash reports are usually prepared at the end of each business day to reflect the sales for that day. Before the cash report can be prepared, all the necessary information must be collected. An opening and closing reading is determined for each cash register. The amount of cash, checks, bank charges, other charges, and paid outs are totaled. Also, all deductions are totaled including coupons, discounts, voids, refunds, and over-rings.

Calculations for the total column should always be double-checked to ensure that the vertical totals equal the horizontal totals.

Following is an example of a cash report for a drugstore/pharmacy with three cash registers

	Reg 1	Reg 2	Reg 3	Total
+ Cash + Checks	1513.12	45.12	2002.02	3560.26
+ Bank Charges	120.00		350.44	470.44
+ House Charges				
+ Paid Outs				
Total	1633.12	45.12	2352.46	4030.70
+ Closing Reading	105060.56	21012.12	210121.12	336193.80
– Opening Reading	103350.54	20967.00	207768.62	332086.16
= Difference	1710.02	45.12	2352.50	4107.64
– Coupons	1.10			1.10
– Discounts	8.90			8.90
– Voids	10.00			10.00
– Refunds				
– Over-rings	56.65			56.65
Total	1633.37	45.12	2352.50	4030.99
+/–	−0.25	0	−0.04	−0.29

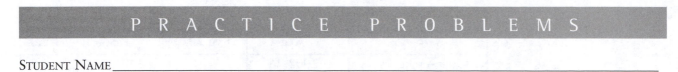

PRACTICE PROBLEMS

STUDENT NAME_____

DATE _____ COURSE NUMBER _____

1. Balance the following cash report:

	Reg 1	Reg 2	Reg 3	Total
+ Cash + Checks	513.12		300.44	
+ Bank Charges	120.00			
+ House Charges			52.02	
+ Paid Outs		5.12		
Total	633.12	5.12	352.46	
+ Closing Reading	105060.56	21062.12	208121.12	
– Opening Reading	104350.54	20967.00	207768.62	
= Difference	710.02	95.12	352.50	
– Coupons				
– Discounts	8.90			
– Voids	10.00			
– Refunds				
– Over-rings	56.65			
Total	634.47	95.12	352.50	
+/–				

2. Balance the following cash report:

	Reg 1	Reg 2	Reg 3	Total
+ Cash + Checks	1145.63		4322.12	
+ Bank Charges	366.12		980.35	
+ House Charges				
+ Paid Outs				
Total				
+ Closing Reading	354632.12		17524.82	
– Opening Reading	353099.50		12222.35	
= Difference				
– Coupons	18.90			
– Discounts				
– Voids				
– Refunds				
– Over-rings				
Total				
+ /–				

3. Balance the following cash report:

	Reg 1	Reg 2	Reg 3	Total
+ Cash + Checks	2002.26		3601.47	
+ Bank Charges	89.12		12.99	
+ House Charges				
+ Paid Outs				
Total				
+ Closing Reading	455325.10		29159.83	
− Opening Reading	453233.55		25543.27	
= Difference				
− Coupons				
− Discounts			1.10	
− Voids				
− Refunds				
− Over-rings				
Total				
+ /−				

4. Find the error in the following cash report, then balance the cash report:

	Reg 1	Reg 2	Reg 3	Total
+ Cash + Checks	1513.12	45.12	2002.02	3560.26
+ Bank Charges	120.00		350.44	470.44
+ House Charges				
+ Paid Outs				
Total	1393.12	45.12	2352.46	4030.70
+ Closing Reading	105060.56	21012.12	210121.12	336193.80
− Opening Reading	103350.54	20967.00	207768.62	332086.16
= Difference	1710.02	45.12	2352.50	4107.64
− Coupons	1.10			1.10
− Discounts	8.90			8.90
− Voids	10.00			10.00
− Refunds				
− Over-rings	56.65			56.65
Total	1633.37	45.12	2352.50	4030.99
+ /−	−240.25	0	−0.04	−0.29

Calculations for Institutional Pharmacy

27 Parenteral Doses Using Ratio and Proportion Calculations

PHARMACY TECHNICIANS PREPARE parenteral medications for use in hospitals, home health care, and long term care. Parenteral medications are medications that are injected into the body by different routes such as:

- IV (intravenous)

- IM (intramuscular)

- SC (subcutaneous)

Parenteral medications are available as liquids and as powders. A drug in powder form must be reconstituted before it can be injected. The strength or concentration of a medication is usually expressed as a measurement of weight (mg, g, units) in a specified volume (ml, cc). For example, 250 mg/ml or 10,000 units/2 cc.

Note: In pharmacy practice, milliliters (ml) and cubic centimeters (cc) are considered interchangeable.

Calculations must be made to convert the measurement of weight ordered by the physician into a volume. Different size syringes are used to measure this volume for injection, either into the patient or into a solution bag for infusion into the patient.

Ratio and Proportion Calculations

Most pharmacy calculations problems can be solved using the ratio and proportion method. A ratio expresses the relationship between two quantities. For example, 250 mg/ml means there are 250 mg of drug in each ml of solution. A proportion is an equation that states that two specific ratios are equal. The equation is written with an equals (=) sign between the two ratios. For example, 1:2 = 3:6 (1:2 is the same as 3:6).

A proportion consists of four terms. If three of the terms are known, then the fourth term (designated as X), can be calculated. When using ratio and proportion to solve a problem, each side of the equation must be set up the same—meaning that all units of measurement must be the same. (Do not mix grams and milligrams or liters and milliliters.) Always label values with the units of measurement. For example:

$$\frac{grams}{milliliters} = \frac{grams}{milliliters} \quad and \quad \frac{mg}{ml} = \frac{mg}{ml}$$

Important: Set up the proportion as ratio of drug available = ratio of drug required. That is, put the known value on the left side and unknown on the right side.

Once a proportion is set up correctly, you can solve the equation by cross multiplying.

Example:

You have on hand a drug with a concentration of 250 mg/ml. How many mg are in 2 ml of the solution?

$$\frac{250 \text{ mg}}{1 \text{ ml}} \searrow = \swarrow \frac{X}{2 \text{ ml}} \rightarrow X \times 1 \text{ ml} = 2 \text{ ml} \times 250 \text{ mg}$$

divide each side by 1 ml and cancel out the units

→ $\dfrac{X \times \cancel{1 \text{ ml}}}{\cancel{1 \text{ ml}}} = \dfrac{2 \text{ ml} \times 250 \text{ mg}}{1 \cancel{ml}}$ → X = 500 mg *answer*

Example:

How many mls are needed for a 500 mg dose of a drug with a concentration of 250 mg/ml?

$$\frac{250 \text{ mg}}{1 \text{ ml}} \searrow = \swarrow \frac{500 \text{ mg}}{X} \rightarrow X \times 250 \text{ mg} = 1 \text{ ml} \times 500 \text{ mg}$$

→ divide each side by 250 mg and cancel out the units

→ $\dfrac{X \times \cancel{250 \text{ mg}}}{\cancel{250 \text{ mg}}} = \dfrac{1 \text{ ml} \times 500 \cancel{mg}}{250 \cancel{mg}}$

→ X 2 ml *answer*

Example:

A doctor orders a 500 mg dose of a medication. The medication is available as 1 gram per 2 ml. How many mls are needed?

Change the grams to milligrams so the units of measurement are the same:

Available 1 g / 2 ml = 1000 mg / 2 ml

Set up a ratio and proportion problem:

$$\frac{1000 \text{ mg}}{2 \text{ ml}} = \frac{500 \text{ mg}}{X} \rightarrow X \times 1000 \text{ mg} = 500 \text{ mg} \times 2 \text{ ml}$$

→ divide both sides by 1000 mg and cancel out the units

→ $\dfrac{X \times \cancel{1000 \text{ mg}}}{\cancel{1000 \text{ mg}}} = \dfrac{500 \cancel{mg} \times 2 \text{ ml}}{1000 \cancel{mg}}$

→ X = 1 ml *answer*

Example:

How many grams of dextrose are in 20 ml of a solution containing 50 g of dextrose in 100 ml of water?

Set up a ratio and proportion problem:

$$\frac{50 \text{ g}}{100 \text{ ml}} = \frac{X}{20 \text{ ml}}$$ ➔ X × 100 ml = 50 g × 20 ml

➔ divide both sides by 100 ml and cancel out the units

➔ $\dfrac{X \times \cancel{100 \text{ ml}}}{\cancel{100 \text{ ml}}} = \dfrac{50\text{g} \times 20 \cancel{\text{ ml}}}{100 \cancel{\text{ ml}}}$

➔ X = 10 g *answer*

PRACTICE PROBLEMS

STUDENT NAME _____

DATE _____   COURSE NUMBER _____

1.   A TPN requires the addition of 15 units of regular insulin U-100. A 10 ml vial of insulin contains 1000 units. How many mls of insulin should be added to the TPN?

2.   You receive an order for heparin 12,000 units in 250 ml D5W. If the strength of the heparin available is 5,000 units/ml, how many mls of heparin do you use?

3.   Calculate the number of milliliters required to prepare the following concentrations:

   a.   25 mEq potassium chloride (stock: 2 mEq/ml KCl)

   b.   37.5 mg methotrexate (stock: methotrexate 50 mg/2 ml)

   c.   1050 mg fluorouracil (stock: fluorouracil 50 mg/ml)

   d.   62.5 mg doxorubicin (stock: doxorubicin 50 mg/25 ml)

e.   Methicillin 2.5 G (stock: methicillin 1 G/2 ml)

f.   Scopolamine 200 mcg (stock: scopolamine 0.4 mg/ml)

g.   Potassium phosphate 17.6 mEq (stock: 4.4 mEq/ml potassium phosphate)

h.   200,000 units penicillin (stock: penicillin 500,000 units/ml)

4.   If there is 20 mg of a drug in 10 ml of solution, how many liters of solution will contain 1 G of the drug?

5.   A vial of penicillin contains 3,000,000 units of the powdered drug. How much diluent is needed to make a solution containing 400,000 units of this drug per cc? (Assume no powder volume.)

6.   You have just added 0.2 ml of folic acid to an IV bag. How many mg of folic acid have you added if the stock solution contains 5 mg folic acid per ml?

7.   Elixir of digoxin contains 50 mcg per ml. How many mcg are in 0.3 ml of the solution?

8.   A physician orders 2.5 mg of theophylline to be given orally to a pediatric patient. If the elixir of theophylline contains 80 mg per tablespoonful, how many mls of the elixir should be administered?

9.   How many mls of vitamin B_{12} injection (1000 mcg/ml) must be added to an IV bag to obtain a dose of 0.5 mg of vitamin B_{12}?

10. A physician orders 0.4 mg of a drug. The label on the vial states that the concentration is 500 mcg per 2 ml. How many mls of the drug should be dispensed?

11. The doctor orders Garamycin 70 mg. A 2 ml vial contains 40 mg/ml. How many mls should be dispensed?

12. 7,500 units of a drug are ordered. On hand is a prefilled disposable syringe containing 10,000 units in 1 ml. How many mls should be used?

13. A dose of 65 units of regular insulin is to be added to a TPN bag. You are to use Humulin R (100 units/ml). How many mls would you add?

14. How many mls would you need for a 400 mg dose of chloramphenicol if you had a vial that contained 1 g per 10 ml?

15. Potassium chloride 30 mEq is to be given in 1000 ml of IV fluid. Available vials contain 40 mEq/20 ml. How many mls of the drug would you use?

16. How many mls of potassium chloride solution (2 mEq/ml) is required to prepare a liter bag of D_5W/0.2% NaCl with 25 mEq KCl?

17. How many mls of aminophyllin solution (500 mg/20 ml) is needed to prepare 350 mg aminophyllin in 100 ml D_5W?

18. Levothyroxine comes in 500 mcg vials. If the powder is diluted with 10 ml of sterile water, how many mls are required to provide 0.1 mg?

19. You receive an order for 0.2 g of Tigan IM. You have a 5 ml vial labeled 100 mg/ml. How many mls are required?

20.   Cleocin IV comes as 600 mg/4 ml. How many mls are needed to make a piggy-back of 750 mg in 100 mls of 0.9% Sodium Chloride Injection?

21.   An injection solution is available in a 2.9 mg/5 ml concentration. A patient's required dose is 5.22 mg in 500 mls 0.9% sodium chloride solution. How many mls of the injection solution are needed?

22.   A drug concentration is 0.05 mg/ml in 5 ml vials. A patient requires a 0.25 mg dose. How many mls are used for this dose?

23.   A single IM dose of 2.4 million units of penicillin G is ordered by the physician. The concentration of the injection suspension is 600,000 units per ml in 1 ml, 2 ml, and 4 ml vials. How many mls of the suspension are required?

24.   Clonidine Injection is available as 10 ml vials containing 100 mcg/ml. A patient order is for 0.2 mg daily in 2 equal doses. How many mls will be needed for each dose?

25.   A patient is given 10.8 mls of phenytoin as a loading dose. Phenytoin is available as 50 mg per ml in 2 ml and 5 ml vials. What is the dose in mg that the patient received?

26. Droperidol is available as a 2.5 mg/ml injection. A patient needs a 4 mg slow IV push. How many mls are used?

27. A drug is available as 120 mcg/0.6 ml. The dose required is 100 mcg per day. How many mls will be drawn?

28. A patient needs 11 million units of a drug in a single dose. The drug is available as 6 million units per ml in a 3 ml vial. How many mls will the patient receive?

29. A patient requires 30 units of oxytocin by IV infusion in 1000 mls of fluid. Oxytocin is available as 10 units per ml. How many mls will the patient need?

30. A patient needs a 1 G dose of streptomycin. The drug is available in a 2.5 ml vial, concentration 400 mg/ml. How many mls does the patient need?

31. A 500 ml TPN needs the addition of 33 mEq of sodium chloride. The label on the vial of concentrated Sodium Chloride Injection has the following information: 30 ml single dose, 234 mg/ml, 4 mEq/ml, and 23.4%. How many mls should be added to the TPN bag?

32.   Digoxin Injection is available in a concentration of 0.5 mg in a 2 ml vial. The physician orders a 150 mcg dose in 150 ml of D_5W. How many mls will the patient need?

33.   Tobramycin Injection is available in a concentration of 80 mg per 2 ml. The patient received 1.5 ml in 100 ml of Normal Saline. What was the dose in mg that the patient received?

34.   Humulin R 78 units are to be added to a 1 liter TPN. The 10 ml vial of Humulin R contains 100 units/ml. How many mls are required?

35.   Morphine sulfate 8 mg is ordered by the physician. The label on the morphine sulfate vial reads 15 mg (1 ml fill in 2 ml size). How many mls will the patient receive?

36.   Atropine Sulfate Injection 0.4 mg per ml is available in the pharmacy. The doctor orders 0.8 mg. How many mls will complete this order?

37.   A patient requires potassium chloride 7 mEq in a 1000 ml bag of Lactated Ringers Solution. The pharmacy has on hand Potassium Chloride for Injection 40 mEq in 20 ml vials. How many mls will be needed in the IV bag?

38.   A patient is ordered Novolin R 54 units. The Novolin R available is 1000 units in a 10 ml vial. How many mls will the patient require?

39.   Aminophyllin Injection is available in a 20 ml vial containing 500 mg (25 mg/ml). The physician orders a dose of 400 mg. How many mls will be needed to fill this order?

40.   500 ml of D_5W with 8,000 units of Heparin is ordered for a patient. A 5 ml vial of Heparin contains 10,000 units per ml. How many mls are needed for this patient?

28 Powdered Drug Preparations

SOME PARENTERAL PRODUCTS have limited stability when in solution, such as antibiotics. These drugs are supplied by manufacturers in powder form. When a powdered drug is to be administered to a patient or added to an infusion bag, it is reconstituted with a recommended diluent, usually Sterile Water for Injection. The antibiotic manufacturer's package insert includes other examples of recommended diluents.

The package insert, and sometimes the vial label, also tell how much diluent to add for reconstitution. The label on the vial will also indicate the amount of powdered drug contained in the vial.

The volume or space that the powdered drug occupies after it is reconstituted is called *powder volume* and is expressed in milliliters. For some drugs, the powder volume is so small that it is negligible. Other drugs have a substantial powder volume, which is always taken into consideration when reconstituting. For example, penicillin has substantial powder volume.

If the entire amount of powdered drug after reconstitution is to be used, then powder volume is not critical. However, if a partial dose is to be used, then powder volume is critical and must be calculated so that the final volume and the concentration are accurate.

Vial Size	Diluent Added	Final Volume	Powder Volume
1. 125 mg	1 ml	1 ml	None (1 ml – 1 ml)
2. 250 mg	0.9 ml	1 ml	0.1 ml (1 ml – 0.9 ml)
3. 500 mg	1.8 ml	2 ml	0.2 ml (2 ml – 1.8 ml)
4. 1 g	3.4 ml	4 ml	0.6 ml (4 ml – 3.4 ml)
5. 2 g	6.8 ml	8 ml	1.2 ml (8 ml – 6.8 ml)

Example:

The powder volume equals final volume minus the diluent added.

Increasing volumes of diluent are added to increasing vial sizes to ensure that sufficient diluent is added for dissolution. Concentrations are expressed as weight per one milliliter—for example, mg/ml, units/ml, g/ml.

Example:

What is the concentration of drug in mg/ml for each of the strengths of drug in the previous chart?

Calculate the concentration by dividing the weight of the drug in the vial by the final volume, and then reducing to milligrams in one milliliter.

1. $\dfrac{125 \text{ mg}}{1 \text{ ml}}$ – 125 mg/ml

2. $\dfrac{250 \text{ mg}}{1 \text{ ml}}$ – 250 mg/ml

3. $\dfrac{500 \text{ mg}}{2 \text{ ml}}$ reduce → $\dfrac{500 \text{ mg/\cancel{2} ml}}{2 \quad \cancel{2}}$ → 250 mg/ml

4. 1 g = 1000 mg → $\dfrac{1000 \text{ mg}}{4 \text{ ml}}$ reduce → $\dfrac{1000 \text{ mg/4ml}}{4}$ → 250 mg/ml

5. 2 g = 2000 mg → $\dfrac{2000 \text{ mg}}{8 \text{ ml}}$ reduce → $\dfrac{2000 \text{ mg/\cancel{8}ml}}{\cancel{8}}$ → 250 mg/ml

Example:

You add 18 ml of Sterile Water for Injection to a vial containing 500 mg of a drug that has a powder volume of 2 ml. What is the concentration of the drug in the solution?

First, find the final volume obtained after reconstitution.

Volume of diluent   = 18 ml

Powder volume   = 2 ml

Final volume   = 20 ml

The amount of drug in the vial = 500 mg

Calculate the concentration =

$\dfrac{\text{amount of drug in vial}}{\text{Final volume}}$ and reduce to mg/ml

$\dfrac{500 \text{ mg}}{20 \text{ ml}}$ reduce → $\dfrac{500 \text{ mg/\cancel{20} ml}}{20 \quad \cancel{20}}$ → 25 mg/ml *answer*

Example:

If 17 ml of Sterile Water for Injection is added to 2 g of drug and the concentration obtained is 100 mg/ml, what is the powder volume of the drug?

Set up a ratio and proportion to calculate the ml of final solution.
Remember all units of measurement must be the same. 2 g = 2000 mg

$\dfrac{100 \text{ mg}}{1 \text{ ml}} = \dfrac{2000 \text{ mg}}{X}$ → $\dfrac{X \times \cancel{100 \text{ mg}}}{\cancel{100 \text{ mg}}} = \dfrac{1 \text{ ml} \times 2000 \cancel{\text{ mg}}}{100 \cancel{\text{ mg}}}$

→ X = 20 ml

The final volume = 20 ml (calculated)
Diluent added   = 17 ml (given)

Powder volume   = Final volume − diluent added
  = 20 ml − 17 ml = 3 ml *answer*

STUDENT NAME

DATE   COURSE NUMBER

1. If 95 ml of Sterile Water for Injection is added to a 10 g bulk powdered drug pharmacy container, the concentration obtained is 100 mg/ml. What is the powder volume of the drug?

2. Using another 10 g vial of the drug in question 1, you want a concentration of 200 mg/ml. How many mls of Sterile Water for Injection should be added? (Use the powder volume calculated in question 1.)

3. The package directions for streptomycin instruct you to add 4.2 ml of Sterile Water for Injection to 1 g of dry powder to give a concentration of 200 mg/ml. What is the powder volume of the streptomycin?

4. You have a vial of penicillin G potassium containing 20,000,000 units. The directions are to add 32 ml of Sterile Water for Injection to reconstitute to a concentration of 500,000 units/ml. What is the powder volume of the penicillin?

5. The directions for a vial containing 500 mg of powdered Rocephin state that the addition of 1.8 ml of Sterile Water for Injection will yield a solution containing 250 mg/ml. What is the powder volume of the drug?

6. If you add 8 ml of Sterile Water for Injection to a vial of 5 MU penicillin that has a powder volume of 2 ml, what is the concentration of the drug in solution?

7. You add 10 ml of Sterile Water for Injection to 1 g of a drug that has a powder volume of 0.8 ml. What is the concentration of the drug in mg/ml in the final solution?

8. If you add 27 ml of diluent to a vial containing 2.5 g of drug that has a powder volume of 3 ml, what will be the concentration of the drug after reconstitution?

9. To prepare 3 G of Unasyn, the package insert states to add 6.4 ml of diluent. The concentration obtained is 375 mg/ml. What is the powder volume of the Unasyn?

10. The directions for reconstitution for a 2 G vial of Claforan state to add 10 ml of Sterile Water for Injection to obtain a concentration of 180 mg/ml. What is the final volume obtained after reconstitution?

11. 10 ml of Sterile Water for Injection is added to a 1 G vial of Mefoxin, giving a 10.5 ml final volume. What is the concentration of the reconstituted powdered Mefoxin?

12.   A 6 G pharmacy bulk package of Fortaz is reconstituted with 26 ml of Sterile Water for Injection. What will be the final concentration of the drug if the powder volume of the Fortaz is 4 ml?

13.   You add 23 ml of Sterile Water for Injection to a 3 G vial of antibiotic that has a powder volume of 3 ml. What is the concentration, in mg/ml, of the reconstituted drug?

14.   A 20 G vial of a powdered drug requires the addition of 36 ml of Sterile Water for Injection to give a concentration of 500 mg/ml. What is the powder volume of the drug?

15.   Using another 20 G vial of the drug in question 14, you need a concentration of 400 mg/ml. How many ml of Sterile Water for Injection do you need to add to the vial?

16.   After adding 20 ml of Sterile Water for Injection to a 4 G vial of powdered drug, the concentration is 325 mg/2 ml. What is the powder volume of the drug?

17.   A 1.5 g vial of antibiotic has a powder volume of 1.4 ml. You need a concentration of 125 mg/ml. How many ml of Sterile Water for Injection will you need to add to obtain this concentration?

18.   Calculate the concentration, in mg/ml, after reconstitution with 19 ml of Sterile Water for Injection, of a 2.75 g vial, if the drug has a powder volume of 2.2 ml.

19.   A technician adds 64 ml of Sterile Water for Injection to a pharmacy bulk bottle of 30 G of antibiotic powder. The antibiotic has a powder volume of 6 ml. Calculate the concentration, in mg/ml, obtained after reconstitution.

20.   If you need a concentration of 250 mg/ml and you have on hand a 5 G vial of antibiotic with a powder volume of 1.6 ml, how many ml of Sterile Water for Injection should you add?

21.   A 2 G vial of a drug has a powder volume of 1.5 ml.

   a.   How many mls of Sterile Water for Injection will you add to obtain a concentration of 125 mg/ml?

   b.   A patient dose is 325 mg. How many mls of the reconstituted solution will you use?

22.   An 8 G vial of a powdered drug requires the addition of 9.8 ml of Sterile Water for Injection to obtain a concentration of 800 mg/ml.

   a.   What is the powder volume of the drug?

   b.   If 2.6 ml of the reconstituted solution is added to a 500 ml bag of D5W, what dose (in G) will the patient receive?

23. A 40 G vial of an antibiotic has a powder volume of 5.2 ml. If 94.8 mls of Sterile Water for Injection are added to the vial, what is the concentration (mg/ml) of the reconstituted solution?

24. A patient is ordered a 130 mg dose of a drug in 50 ml of D_5W. A vial contains 1 G of the powdered drug. The drug has a powder volume of 0.4 ml.

   a. How many mls of Sterile Water for Injection are needed to obtain a concentration of 250 mg/ml?

   b. How many mls will be needed to fill the patient order?

25. A 2 G vial of a powdered drug is reconstituted with 100 mls of Sterile Water for Injection. The drug has a powder volume of 2.3 ml. What is the concentration of the reconstituted solution?

26. 10,000,000 units of a powdered antibiotic are contained in a vial. A concentration of 500,000 units per ml is obtained when Sterile Water for Injection is added. The drug has a powder volume of 3.2 ml. How many mls of Sterile Water for Injection should be added to the vial?

27. Using another vial of the antibiotic used in question 26, if 36.8 ml of Sterile Water for Injection is added to the vial what is the concentration of the reconstituted solution?

28.   A 1 G vial of Nafcillin is reconstituted with 3.4 ml of Sterile Water for Injection. A concentration of 250 mg/ml Nafcillin is obtained.

   a.   What is the powder volume of the Nafcillin?

   b.   If a patient requires a 200 mg dose in 250 ml of D_5W, how many mls of the reconstituted solution are needed?

29.   A powdered drug is available in vials containing 35 mg of the drug. The reconstitution instructions indicate to add 6.2 ml of Sterile Water for Injection to obtain a concentration of 5 mg/ml.

   a.   What is the powder volume of the drug?

   b.   How many mls of the reconstituted drug are needed for a 2.5 mg dose in 50 mls NS?

30.   1 ml of Sterile Water for Injection is added to a 1.5 mg vial of a powdered drug with a powder volume of 0.2 ml. What is the concentration in mg/ml of the solution obtained?

31.   A vial contains two different drugs. Medication A: 3.5 mg and medication B: 35 mg. The two drugs together have a powder volume of 0.5 ml. What is the concentration of each medication if 3 ml of Sterile Water for Injection is added to the vial?

32. What is the powder volume of 40 G of a drug if after adding 89.6 ml of Sterile Water for Injection the concentration obtained is 400 mg/ml?

33. A physician has ordered a loading dose of 600 mg in 50 ml of Normal Saline. The powder volume of the drug ordered is 0.9 ml.

    a. How many mls of Sterile Water for Injection must be added to the 5 G vial of drug to obtain a concentration of 250 mg/ml?

    b. How many mls of the reconstituted solution are needed for the patient's dose?

34. A 9 G vial of powdered medication is reconstituted with Sterile Water for Injection to a concentration of 300 mg/ml. How many mls of SWFI should be added if the powder volume of the drug is 1.3 ml?

35. What is the concentration in G/ml of 35 G of a drug with a powder volume of 4 mls if 31 mls of Sterile Water for Injection are added to the vial?

36. A patient requires 250 mcg of a medication in 50 ml of D$_5$W. A 4 mg vial of the medication has a powder volume of 0.1 ml 3.9 mls of Sterile Water for Injection is added to the vial.

    a. What is the final concentration of the reconstituted solution?

    b. How many mls does the patient need?

37.   A 1.5 G vial of Unasyn contains two drugs: 1 G ampicillin and 0.5 G of sulbactam. The powder volume of the Unasyn is 0.8 ml. The label instructions indicate that 3.2 ml of SWI should be used to reconstitute the drug. What is the concentration of each of the drugs?

38.   A drug concentration of 250 mg/ml is needed. The powdered drug is available in a 10 G vial with a powder volume of 2.4 ml. How many mls of Sterile Water for Injection should be added to the vial to obtain the needed concentration?

39.   A physician orders for a patient 8 MU of a drug in 100 mls of 0.9% sodium chloride solution. The drug is available as a 20 MU powder for reconstitution with Sterile Water for Injection. The instructions are to add 32 mls of SWI to obtain a concentration of 500,000 units/ml.

        a.   What is the powder volume of the drug?

        b.   How many mls of the reconstituted solution will the patient need?

40.   If 7.2 mls of SWI are added to 16 G of powdered medication with a powder volume of 0.8 ml, what is the final concentration in G/ml of the reconstituted solution?

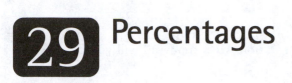

Percentages

THE STRENGTHS OF MANY SOLUTIONS are expressed as a percentage. For example, 0.9% Sodium Chloride Injection; 5% Dextrose Injection. A solution is composed of two parts—the solute and the solvent:

- The solvent is the substance (usually a liquid, but it can be a solid) in which the solute is dissolved.

- The solute is the substance dissolved by the solvent. The percentage strength of pharmaceutical compounds is represented by a given weight, in grams, of a drug (solute) in 100 ml of solution (solvent). For example, 1 g in 100 ml = 1%; 15 g in 100 ml = 15%.

- Dextrose Injection 5% (D_5W) contains 5 grams of dextrose per 100 ml of solution: 5 g/100 ml;

$$\frac{5g}{100 \text{ ml}}$$

- Sodium Chloride Injection 0.9% (Normal Saline) contains 0.9 grams of sodium chloride per 100 ml solution: 0.9 g/100ml;

$$\frac{0.9g}{100 \text{ ml}}$$

- Concentrated Sodium Chloride Solution 23.4% contains 23.4 g of sodium chloride per 100 ml of solution: 23.4 g/100 ml;

$$\frac{23.4 \text{ g}}{100 \text{ ml}}$$

Some parenteral medications are expressed as a percentage strength. For example:

- Magnesium Sulfate Injection 50%

- Calcium Gluconate Injection 10%

- Potassium Acetate Injection 19.6%

If a physician orders a dose in milligrams or grams, calculations can be made from the percentage strength concentrations.

Example:

Iodine tincture is available as a 2% solution of iodine. How many grams of iodine will be contained in 40 ml of the tincture?

$$2\% = \frac{2 \text{ g}}{100 \text{ ml}}$$

Set up a ratio and proportion using the above value

$$\frac{2 \text{ g}}{100 \text{ ml}} = \frac{X}{40 \text{ ml}} \rightarrow X \times \cancel{100 \text{ ml}} = \frac{2 \text{ g} \times 40 \cancel{\text{ ml}}}{100 \cancel{\text{ml}}} \rightarrow X = 0.8 \text{ g } answer$$

Example:

You have 25 grams of a drug and need to compound a 30% solution. How many ml will you be able to prepare?

$$30\% = \frac{30\ g}{100\ ml}$$

Set up a ratio and proportion problem using the above value.

$$\frac{30\ g}{100\ ml} = \frac{25\ g}{X} \;\rightarrow\; \frac{X \times \cancel{30\ g}}{\cancel{30\ g}} = \frac{100\ ml \times 25\ \cancel{g}}{30\ \cancel{g}} \;\rightarrow\; X = 83.3\ ml\ \textit{answer}$$

Example:

You add 80 grams of a drug to 600 ml of sterile water. What is the percentage strength of the solution prepared? Remember percentage is grams in 100 ml.

To find the percentage, find the number of grams in 100 ml.

Set up a ratio and proportion problem:

$$\frac{80\ g}{600\ ml} = \frac{X}{100\ ml} \;\rightarrow\; \frac{X \times \cancel{600\ ml}}{\cancel{600\ ml}} = \frac{80\ g \times 100\ \cancel{ml}}{600\ \cancel{ml}} \;\rightarrow\; X = 13.3\ g$$

$$\rightarrow\; 13.3\%\ \textit{answer}$$

There is an alternative method for solving the previous question:

$$\text{Known ratio} = \frac{80\ g}{600\ ml}$$

To find percentage multiply by 100 $\rightarrow \;\dfrac{80\ g}{600\ ml} \times 100 = 13.3\%\ \textit{answer}$

Example:

You have an order for 2 g of calcium gluconate to add to a 1000 ml bag of 5% Dextrose Injection. The label on the calcium gluconate vial gives the concentration as 10% and 0.465 mEq/ml. How many ml will you need to use? Remember: Do not mix units.

To calculate the 2 g dose, you will use the 10% concentration, *not* the mEq/ml concentration.

Set up a ratio and proportion problem using 10% = 10 g in 100 ml.

$$\frac{10\ g}{100\ ml} = \frac{2\ g}{X} \;\rightarrow\; \frac{X \times \cancel{10\ g}}{\cancel{10\ g}} = \frac{100\ ml \times 2\ \cancel{g}}{10\ \cancel{g}} \;\rightarrow\; X = 20\ ml\ \textit{answer}$$

PRACTICE PROBLEMS

STUDENT NAME _____

DATE _____ COURSE NUMBER _____

1. How many G of amino acid are in 500 ml of 8.5% solution?

2. What percent strength solution would result if you mixed 3 G of NaCl in enough water to make 25 ml?

3. A powdered drug comes in a vial containing 2.4 G. If the total volume after the diluent is injected is 6 ml, what is the percent strength of the solution?

4. A patient medication order calls for a liter bottle of acetic acid irrigation solution 0.25%. How many mg of acetic acid are contained in each 30 ml irrigation dose?

5. You have dissolved 170 G of a drug in 1 liter of water. What is the percentage strength of the solution formed?

6. You have dissolved 13.5 g of a drug in 500 ml of sterile water. What is the percentage strength of the solution prepared?

7.   On hand is a 50 ml vial of mannitol injection 25%. The order requires 3.5 G. How many mls should be withdrawn from the vial?

8.   How many mg of zinc sulfate are found in 4 oz. of a 0.02% solution?

9.   A solution of ampicillin contains 250 mg/ml. Calculate the percentage strength of the solution.

10.   How many grams of glucose are contained in 1500 ml of a 10% glucose solution?

11.   How many grams of a drug are contained in 500 ml of a 20% solution?

12.   How many grams of mercuric chloride are required to prepare 250 ml of a 5% solution?

13.   How many mg of certified red color should be used in preparing 5 liters of a 0.01% solution?

14.   How many mls of a 4% stock solution of silver nitrate contain 150 mg of silver nitrate?

15.   How many grams of pure drug are used in preparing 250 ml of a 0.5% solution?

16.   How many mg of potassium chloride are in one tablespoonful of a 10% KCl solution?

17.   How many 150 mg clindamycin capsules are needed to prepare 60 ml of a 1% clindamycin solution?

18.   A patient is to be given 2 G of magnesium sulfate IM. The label on a 10 ml vial reads "50% solution of Mag Sulf." How many ml will you need?

19.   You have 30 ml of 1% lidocaine on the shelf. The order calls for 40 mg. How many ml do you need to use?

20.   You have 150 mg of cocaine to prepare a 0.4% cocaine solution. How many ml will you be able to prepare?

21.   You need to prepare 150 G of a 2% zinc oxide ointment. How many grams of zinc oxide powder will be needed to prepare this ointment?

22.   The pharmacy has on hand 1000 ml of an 8% sodium chloride Solution. How many grams of sodium chloride are in the solution?

23.   A technician receives an order to prepare 250 ml of a 32% sodium chloride solution. How many grams of sodium chloride crystals will the technician weigh?

24.   A 0.3% potassium permanganate solution is ordered for a patient. The physician orders 60 mls. How many mg of potassium permanganate are needed?

25.   An order is received in the pharmacy for 500 G of a 27% antibiotic ointment. How many grams of the antibiotic powder will be needed to make this ointment?

26.   You have on hand 500 mg of a powder. How many mls of 2% solution can you prepare?

27.   There are 24 G of sodium chloride crystals in the pharmacy. How many liters of a 1/2% solution can the technician prepare?

28. An order is sent to the pharmacy for 1.5 L of a 1/4% solution. How many grams of the powdered drug must be used?

29. A technician is asked to prepare 60 mls of an 80% solution. How many grams of the solid must be weighed?

30. You have in stock a 30 ml vial of 23.4% concentrated Sodium Chloride Injection.

    a.   How many grams of sodium chloride are in the vial?

    b.   How many mg are in 1 ml?

31. Calcium Gluconate is available as a 10% solution. An order is for 1.5 G of calcium gluconate. How many mls of the solution should be used?

32. Hydrocortisone topical cream is available as a 0.2% concentration in 454 G. How many milligrams of hydrocortisone are in the product?

33. Devonex is a topical ointment available in a 0.005% concentration. How many mg of the active ingredient are contained in 60 G?

34.   You have 25 mg of chloramphenicol powder in the pharmacy. How many ml of a 1% ophthalmic solution will you be able to prepare?

35.   You have dissolved 8.8 G of a powder in 160 mls of solvent. What is the percentage strength of the solution?

36.   The label on a 10 ml vial of a drug indicates a concentration of 4 mg/ml. Express this as a percentage strength.

37.   Co-Trimoxazole Injection contains sulfamethoxazole 80 mg and trimethoprim 16 mg per ml in 50 ml vials. What are the percentage strengths of each of the drugs?

38.   Co-Trimoxazole oral suspension contains sulfamethoxazole 200 mg and trimethoprim 40 mg per 5 ml. The suspension is available in 200 ml bottles. What are the percentage strengths of the two drugs?

39.   You need to prepare 60 mls of a 0.025% solution. How many mg of powder will you need to dissolve?

40.   A liter bag of dextrose solution contains 450 G of dextrose. What is the percentage strength of the dextrose solution?

30 Ratio Solutions

THE STRENGTH of weak pharmaceutical solutions is sometimes expressed as a ratio. A ratio is a comparison of one quantity to another similar quantity. The quantities that are compared are referred to as the terms of the ratio. The terms of the ratio are written with a colon (:) between them. You will see concentrations such as 1:1000 and 1:10,000. They can also be expressed as a fraction. For example:

$$1:1000 \rightarrow \frac{1}{1000}$$

Percentages are ratios of parts per 100. For example, 5% means 5 parts per 100, or when expressed as a ratio 5:100 (said 5 in 100).

Ratio strengths are usually reduced to their lowest terms, so the first number in the ratio is a 1. To reduce a ratio where the first number is not a 1, divide both terms of the ratio by the value of the first number. For example:

5:100 can be reduced by dividing each side of the ratio by 5

$$\frac{5}{5} : \frac{100}{5} \rightarrow 1:20 \ (1 \text{ in } 20)$$

4:1000 can be reduced by dividing each side of the ratio by 4

$$4:1000 \rightarrow \frac{4}{4} : \frac{1000}{4} \rightarrow 1:250 \ (1 \text{ in } 250)$$

Ratios can be converted to percentages by changing the ratio to a fraction and multiplying by 100.

$$1:20 \rightarrow \frac{1}{20} \times 100 = 5\%$$

$$1:25 \rightarrow \frac{1}{25} \times 100 = 4\%$$

$$1:1000 \rightarrow \frac{1}{1000} \times 100 = 0.1\%$$

$$1:20,000 \rightarrow \frac{1}{20,000} \times 100 = 0.005\%$$

When a ratio is used to express the concentration of a pharmaceutical compound, it is interpreted as follows:

- Solids in liquids are weight in volume solutions (w/v)

- Liquids in liquids are volume in volume solutions (v/v)

- Solids in solids are weight in weight compounds (w/w)

Using 1:1000 as an example:

- a w/v solution will contain 1 g in 1000 ml of solution (1:1000 w/v)

- a v/v solution will contain 1 ml in 1000 ml of solution (1:1000 v/v)

- a w/w compound will contain 1 g in 1000 g of compound (1:1000 w/w)

Using 1:20 as an example:

- a w/v solution will contain 1 g in 20 ml of solution (1:20 w/v)

- a v/v solution will contain 1 ml in 20 ml of solution (1:20 v/v)

- a w/w compound will contain 1 g in 20 g of compound (1:20 w/w)

Example:

How many grams of sodium bicarbonate are needed to make 200 ml of a 1:1000 w/v solution?

1:1000 w/v means 1 g in 1000 ml.

Set up a ratio and proportion problem as follows:

$$\frac{1\ g}{1000\ ml} = \frac{X}{200\ ml} \;\rightarrow\; \frac{X \times 1000\ ml}{1000\ ml} = \frac{1\ g \times 200\ ml}{1000\ ml} \;\rightarrow\; X = 0.2\ g\ \textit{answer}$$

Example:

How many ml of boric acid solution will be required to prepare 1000 ml of a 1:20 v/v solution?

1:20 v/v means 1 ml in 20 ml

Set up a ratio and proportion problem as follows:

$$\frac{1\ ml}{20\ ml} = \frac{X}{1000\ ml} \;\rightarrow\; \frac{X \times 20\ ml}{20\ ml} = \frac{1\ ml \times 1000\ ml}{20\ ml} \;\rightarrow\; X = 50\ ml\ \textit{answer}$$

STUDENT NAME _____

DATE _____ COURSE NUMBER _____

1. You are to prepare 2 L of 1:1000 w/v Neosporin bladder irrigation. How many G of Neosporin are required?

2. A 1000 ml of a 1:10 w/v sodium hypochlorite solution is ordered. How many G of sodium hypochlorite do you need to weigh?

3. How many ml of a drug solution are needed to prepare 2.5 L of a 1:20 v/v solution?

4. You need to prepare 750 ml of a 1:500 w/v potassium permanganate solution. How many G are needed?

5. Neostigmine is available in a 1:1000 concentration in a 20 ml vial. The patient order is for 12.5 mg. How many ml are required?

6. What is the percentage strength of a 1:60 solution?

7. How many mg of boric acid are needed to make 150 mls of 1:400 w/v solution of boric aid?

8. A prescription requires 80 mg of cocaine. On the shelf is a 1:40 w/v solution of cocaine. How many ml are needed for this prescription?

9. How many G of potassium permanganate are required to prepare 500 ml of a 1:2500 w/v solution of potassium permanganate?

10. You are asked to make 500 ml of a 1:10,000 w/v gentian violet solution. How many mg of the gentian violet will you need to weigh?

11. Express 0.01% as a ratio.

12. If 150 mg of ascorbic acid powder are mixed with 7.35 g of lactose, what is the ratio strength of ascorbic acid to lactose in the mixture?

13. An order reads Adrenalin 0.4 mg SC q3h prn for asthma. Adrenalin is available in 1 ml ampoules of adrenalin 1:1000. How many ml are needed for a single dose?

14.   How many mg of lidocaine and epinephrine are in 20 ml of lidocaine
        1% and epinephrine 1:100,000?

15.   Calculate the milligrams of drug needed to prepare 400 g of a
        1:2500 w/w ointment.

16.   A technician is required to prepare 20 G of a 1:10,000 w/w ointment.
        How many mg of the drug are needed?

17.   Epinephrine is available as 1:1000 w/v solution. If the patient dose is
        0.1 mg IM, how many ml are needed?

18.   Bupivicaine is available as a 1:400 w/v solution. The patient is given
        10 ml. How many milligrams of bupivicaine did the patient receive?

19.   A 1:50,000 lidocaine solution is to be given to a patient. What is the
        concentration of the solution in mcg/ml?

20.   A technician is to add 1.2 mg of a drug to a 25 ml bag of 5%
        Dextrose Injection. On hand is a 2 ml ampoule of a 1:1000 w/v
        solution. How many ml should be added to the bag?

21.   Adrenalin Injection is available in 1 ml ampoules with a strength of 1:1000 w/v. What is the strength in mg/ml?

22.   Adrenalin Injection is also available as a 1:100,000 w/v strength. Express this concentration in mcg/ml.

23.   What is the percentage strength of a 1:100,000 w/v solution?

24.   A patient is to receive a medication dose of 0.5 mg in 50 ml of Normal Saline of a 1:1000 w/v solution. How many mls will be needed for this dose?

25.   You are to prepare 30 mls of a 1:400 w/v solution. How many mg of powdered drug will you use to make the solution?

26.   A technician adds 40 mg of potassium permanganate crystals to 500 mls of distilled water. What is the ratio strength (w/v) of the solution obtained?

27.   A patient is to receive 5 ml of a 1:2000 w/v solution. How many mg of the drug in the solution will the patient receive?

28. Express 1:2000 w/v as a percentage.

29. Express 0.025% as a w/v ratio.

30. A drug is available in 10 ml multiple dose vials in a concentration of 100 mcg/ml.

   a. What is the w/v ratio strength of the solution?

   b. What is the percentage strength of the solution?

31. A technician receives an order in the pharmacy for 750 mls of a 1:4000 w/v solution. How many mg will be needed to make this solution?

32. On hand in the pharmacy is 14 G of a drug in powder form. The technician is asked to use the 14 G to make a 1:5000 w/v solution. How many liters will the technician be able to prepare?

33. An order for 1 liter of a 1:4000 w/v solution is received in the pharmacy. In stock is 270 mg of the powdered drug. Will the technician be able to fill this order?

34.   A 2:10,000 w/v solution is available. What is the percentage strength of this solution?

35.   A patient requires a 100 mcg dose of a drug which is available as a 1:1000 w/v solution. How many mls of the solution will be added to a 50 ml bag of 0.9% Sodium Chloride Injection to fill the patient order?

36.   An order is received in the pharmacy for 50 mls of a 1:100,000 w/v solution. How many mcg are needed to fill this order?

37.   How many grams of a drug are needed to prepare 550 G of a 1:250 w/w ointment?

38.   A patient is ordered 125 mg of a drug in 500 mls of D5W solution. The concentration of the drug solution available is 1:200 w/v. How many mls of the solution will be added to the bag?

39.   A drug solution is labeled 1:50 w/v. What is the percentage strength of the solution?

40.   A technician is to prepare 150 mls of a 1:2000 w/v solution. How many mg of the drug required will be needed to prepare the solution?

31 Dosage Calculations Based on Body Weight

THE BODY WEIGHT OF A PATIENT is used in calculating accurate doses of medications, especially for pediatric and geriatric patients and also for potent drugs such as chemotherapy agents. This method of calculation is considered more reliable than doses based on age. Doses are expressed as milligrams per kilogram (Kg) or micrograms per kilogram or milligrams per pound of body weight: mg/Kg or mcg/Kg or mg/lb. Conversions from pounds to kilograms or kilograms to pounds must be made when necessary. The conversion factor is 1 kilogram (Kg) = 2.2 pounds (lbs.).

Example:

A patient weighs 121 pounds. What is her weight in kilograms?

1 Kg = 2.2 lb.

Set up a ratio and proportion problem.

$$\frac{1 \text{ Kg}}{2.2 \text{ lb.}} = \frac{X}{121 \text{ lb.}} \;\rightarrow\; \frac{X \times 2.2 \text{ lb.}}{2.2 \text{ lb.}} = \frac{1 \text{ Kg} \times 121 \text{ lb.}}{2.2 \text{ lb.}} \;\rightarrow\; X = 55 \text{ Kg } answer$$

Example:

A patient weighs 90 Kg. The dosage is based on mg/lb. body weight. What does this patient weigh in pounds?

1 Kg = 2.2 lb.

Set up a ratio and proportion.

$$\frac{1 \text{ Kg}}{2.2 \text{ lb.}} = \frac{90 \text{ Kg}}{X} \;\rightarrow\; \frac{X \times 1 \text{ Kg}}{1 \text{ Kg}} = \frac{90 \text{ Kg} \times 2.2 \text{ lb.}}{1 \text{ Kg}} \;\rightarrow\; X = 198 \text{ lb. } answer$$

Example:

A pediatric patient is ordered a 2 mg/Kg single dose of a chemotherapy drug. The child weighs 44 pounds. How many mg will the child receive in the single dose?

Convert the weight from pounds to kilograms: ➜ 1 Kg = 2.2 lb.

$$\frac{1 \text{ Kg}}{2.2 \text{ lb.}} = \frac{X}{44 \text{ lb.}} \;\rightarrow\; \frac{X \times 2.2 \text{ lb.}}{2.2 \text{ lb.}} = \frac{1 \text{ Kg} \times 44 \text{ lb.}}{2.2 \text{ lb.}} \;\rightarrow\; X = 20 \text{ Kg}$$

The dose is 2 mg/Kg.

Set up a ratio and proportion.

$$\frac{2 \text{ mg}}{1 \text{ Kg}} = \frac{X}{20 \text{ Kg}} \;\rightarrow\; \frac{X \times 1 \text{ Kg}}{1 \text{ Kg}} = \frac{2 \text{ mg} \times 20 \text{ Kg}}{1 \text{ Kg}} \;\rightarrow\; X = 40 \text{ mg } answer$$

Example:

An infant weighs 6 pounds. The dose of vancomycin to be given is 15 mg/Kg/day divided into two doses. What is the dose, in mg, for one dose?

Convert 6 lb. to Kg → 1 Kg = 2.2 lb.

Set up a ratio and proportion:

$$\frac{1 \text{ Kg}}{2.2 \text{ lb.}} = \frac{X}{6 \text{ lb.}} \quad \rightarrow \quad \frac{X \times \cancel{2.2 \text{ lb.}}}{\cancel{2.2 \text{ lb.}}} = \frac{1 \text{ Kg} \times 6 \cancel{\text{ lb.}}}{2.2 \cancel{\text{ lb.}}} \quad \rightarrow \quad X = 2.7 \text{ Kg}$$

The dose is 15 mg for each Kg per day.

Set up a ratio and proportion:

$$\frac{15 \text{ mg}}{1 \text{ Kg}} = \frac{X}{2.7 \text{ Kg}} \quad \rightarrow \quad \frac{X \times \cancel{1 \text{ Kg}}}{\cancel{1 \text{ Kg}}} = \frac{15 \text{ mg} \times 2.7 \cancel{\text{ Kg}}}{1 \cancel{\text{ Kg}}}$$

→ X = 40.5 mg per day

The vancomycin is divided into two doses.

40.5 mg/2 = 20.25 mg per dose. *answer*

Doses in milliliters, for addition to infusions, can then be calculated using the concentration found on the vial label of the particular drug ordered by the physician.

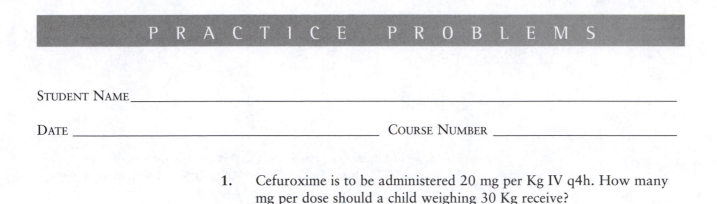

STUDENT NAME_____

DATE _____ COURSE NUMBER _____

1. Cefuroxime is to be administered 20 mg per Kg IV q4h. How many mg per dose should a child weighing 30 Kg receive?

2. A physician orders a medication available as 500 mg tablets for a 110-pound patient. The recommended dose for the drug is 20 mg/Kg per dose. How many tablets should be given to the patient for each dose?

3. The doctor orders vancomycin 10 mg/Kg q12h IV for a newborn. The infant weighs 4000 g. How many mg should be given per dose?

4. A physician orders cyclophosphamide to be given 5 mg/Kg qid in 50ml D_5W. The patient weighs 132 pounds. If the concentration of the drug available is 500 mg/10 ml, how many ml should be added to each bag?

5. A physician requests an aminophyllin infusion. The order is for 1000 mg aminophyllin in 500 ml of D_5W. If the patient weighs 182 pounds and is to receive 0.6 mg/Kg, how many ml will deliver the required dose?

6. An adult intravenous dose of zidovudine is 2 mg/Kg every four hours six times daily. How many mg will a 180-pound patient receive daily?

7. The dose of vincristine, based on the patient's body weight, is 25 mcg/Kg. The drug is available as 500 mcg/ml. The patient weighs 110 pounds. How many ml are used for a dose?

8. A patient weighs 44 pounds and is receiving ampicillin at a rate of 100 mg/Kg/day. What is the total daily dose in grams?

9. Calculate a single dose, in milliliters, for a 20-pound child receiving gentamicin 2 mg/Kg of body weight IVPB q8h. Gentamicin is available in 20 mg/2 ml concentration.

10. Immune globulin is available in a concentration of 6g /100 ml. The order for a 55-pound child is 0.2 g/Kg IV. How many ml are needed for this dose?

11. A 26-pound child is to receive ampicillin at a dose of 50 mg/Kg/day in four equally divided doses. The ampicillin is available in a concentration of 125 mg/5 ml. How many ml are needed for one dose?

12.   A medication order for a patient weighing 154 pounds calls for 0.25 mg of amphotericin B per Kg of body weight to be added to 500 ml of 5% Dextrose Injection. If the amphotericin B is to be obtained from a 10 ml vial containing 50 mg, how many mls should be added to the Dextrose Injection?

13.   The infusion rate for theophylline for acute bronchospasm is 0.5 mg/Kg/hour. How many mg of the drug will the patient receive in 24 hours, if the body weight of the patient is 100 pounds?

14.   A physician orders a drug 5 mg/Kg three times a day for one week. What is the total daily dose, in grams, for a patient weighing 120 pounds?

15.   A 160-pound man is admitted to the hospital. The order states that the patient is to receive 7.5 mg/Kg of acyclovir in 1000 mls of D_5W over 24 hours. The drug comes in 500 mg vials, which are diluted with 10 ml of sterile water (assume no powder volume). How many ml are to be added to the bag?

16.   A pediatrician has prescribed penicillin VK oral suspension for a 66-pound patient. The prescription states that the patient is to receive 50,000 units/Kg/day in four equal divided doses for 10 days. On the shelf is penicillin VK 250mg/5ml (1500 units penicillin VK/mg). How many ml are needed for one dose?

17.   A five year old child weighing 45 pounds is to be given an oral dose of Tylenol Elixir. The literature states that a child of this age and weight should not exceed 71 mg/Kg per day. If this daily maximum is to be divided into six doses, how much is each dose in mg? Tylenol Elixir contains 120 mg/5 ml. How many ml are needed for each of the six doses to be given?

18.   A 176-pound patient requires a dose of 5 mcg/Kg/min of dopamine. How many mg will the patient receive in 20 minutes?

19.   A physician orders a bolus dose of a chemotherapy drug at a rate of 2 mg/Kg. The patient weighs 200 pounds. The syringe is labeled 100 mg/5 ml. How many ml are needed for the bolus dose?

20.   A patient weighs 130 pounds. The physician orders gentamicin at 3 mg/Kg per day in three 50 ml piggyback bags. How many mg will be added to each bag?

21.   Gentamycin is ordered 1.5 mg/Kg/dose for a patient who weighs 135 pounds. Gentamycin is available in a 1 ml vial with a concentration of 40 mg/ml. How many mls of Gentamycin should the patient receive?

22.   A patient is to receive a drug IM 0.6 mg/Kg every 4 hours as needed. The patient weighs 28 pounds. The drug concentration is 25 mg/ml. How many mls will the patient need per dose?

23.   A 64-pound child is to receive 300 mg/Kg/day divided into 4 equal doses. The concentration of the drug solution available is 500 mg per ml. How many mls will the child receive for each dose?

24.   A physician writes an order for a 52 pound child for 400,000 units/Kg/day in divided doses every 6 hours. Each dose is administered in a 50 ml bag of D_5W IVPB. The drug is available as 500,000 units per ml. How many mls will be used in each IVPB?

25.   A patient, weighing 80 pounds, is ordered phenobarbital 5 mg/Kg at bedtime. The Phenobarbital Injection Solution is available in 1 ml vials with a concentration of 65 mg/ml. How many mls will the patient need for this dose?

26.   An order is received in the pharmacy for a 172-pound patient for an IV infusion of 5 mcg/Kg/day in 100ml NS. The ordered drug is available in a concentration of 300 mcg/ml in 1 ml or 1.6 ml vials. How many mls will the patient receive per day?

27.   Insulin is available in a concentration of 100 units/ml. A patient order reads 0.8 units/Kg/day in divided doses. The patient weighs 102 pounds How many mls should the patient receive each day?

28.   A neonate weighs 3 1/2 pounds. She is ordered a medication dose of 20 mg/Kg every 12 hours. The medication is available in a concentration of 33.3 mg/ml. How many mls will the infant require per 12 hours?

29.   Succinylcholine is available in a concentration of 20 mg/ml in a 10 ml vial. The order reads 40 mcg/Kg every 5 to 10 minutes as a maintenance dose for the patient who weighs 190 pounds. How many mls will the patient receive for each dose?

30.   The drug ordered is available in the pharmacy in a concentration of 0.5 mg/ml. The physician orders a dose of 25 mcg/Kg for a patient who weighs 160 pounds. How many mls will be needed to fill the order?

31.   Herceptin is ordered as follows:

Dose 1:   4 mg/Kg/week (1st week)
Dose 2, 3, 4 :   2 mg/Kg/week (2nd, 3rd, and 4th week)

The patient weighs 70 Kg. How many mg of Herceptin has the patient received after 4 weeks?

32.   A physician orders a medication for a patient who weighs 130 pounds The order reads 300 mg/Kg in 50 ml D_5W q4h. How many grams of the medication will the patient receive in 24 hours?

33.   A patient order is for 1.5 G/Kg by slow infusion. The patient weighs 145 pounds. The drug concentration is 40 G/150 ml. How many mls will the patient need?

34. A patient needs 4400 units/Kg/hour of a drug for a 12-hour infusion. The patient weighs 172 pounds. What is the total number of units the patient will receive over the 12-hour infusion?

35. Zinc Sulfate Injection is available in a concentration of 1 mg/ml. An order is received in the pharmacy for a five year old child who weighs 49 pounds. The order reads 100 mcg/Kg per day. How many mls will the child receive in one day?

36. A patient is to receive a course of treatment over 3 days. The patient weighs 122 pounds. The dosage is as follows:

    Day 1: 10 mg/Kg
    5 mg/Kg 6 hours later
    Day 2, 3: 5 mg/Kg

    What is the total amount of drug in grams that the patient will need over the course of the treatment?

37. Ceftazidime is ordered for a 52-pound patient at a dosage of 50 mg/Kg/dose every 8 hours. The drug in solution is available in a concentration of 100 mg/ml. How many mls are required for each dose?

38. The dose for a newborn is 800 mg/Kg/day as a continuous infusion. The infant weighs 7.5 pounds. The drug is available as a 100 mg/ml solution. How many mls are needed for the dose?

39.   A drug is available as 39.55 mg/ml in a 10 ml vial. The patient order received in the pharmacy is for 35 mg/Kg/day. The patient weighs 109 pounds. How many mls are required to fill the order?

40.   A 139-pound patient is ordered a medication dose of 125 mg/Kg/ 24 hours. The concentration of the medication to be used is 425 mg/2 ml. How many mls are needed for the patient dose?

32 Dosage Calculations Based on Body Surface Area

BODY SURFACE AREA (BSA) is used to accurately calculate doses for patients receiving chemotherapy agents. BSA is expressed as square meters (m^2). Body surface area is calculated using patient body weight and height, and can be determined by referring to a standard nomogram.

A nomogram has three columns:

- Height (expressed in centimeters and in inches)
- Body surface area (expressed in square meters)
- Weight (expressed in kilograms and in pounds)

The height and weight of the patient are found on the nomogram and then a straight line is drawn connecting the two values. The BSA for that patient is found where the line intersects the BSA column. Many manufacturers of chemotherapy drugs supply BSA calculators with sliding scales. The principle of finding the BSA is similar to the nomogram.

Example:

A physician orders a chemotherapy drug in a dose of 5 mg/m^2. If the patient has a BSA of 2.1 m^2, what will be the dose in mg?

Set up a ratio and proportion

$$\frac{5 \text{ mg}}{1 \text{ m}^2} = \frac{X}{2.1 \text{ m}^2} \rightarrow \frac{X \times 1 \text{ m}^2}{1 \text{ m}^2} = \frac{5 \text{ mg} \times 2.1 \text{ m}^2}{1 \text{ m}^2} \rightarrow X = 10.5 \text{ mg } answer$$

Example:

The physician orders a drug for a child with a BSA of 0.95 m^2. The drug dose is 750 mcg/m^2. What will be the dose in milligrams for this child?

Set up a ratio and proportion:

$$\frac{750 \text{ mcg}}{1 \text{ m}^2} = \frac{X}{0.95 \text{ m}^2} \rightarrow \frac{X \times 1 \text{ m}^2}{1 \text{ m}^2} = \frac{750 \text{ mcg} \times 0.95 \text{ m}^2}{1 \text{ m}^2} \rightarrow X = 712.5 \text{ mcg}$$

The dose is in mg   1 mg = 1000 mcg

To find the number of milligrams, divide the micrograms by 1000.

$$\frac{712.5 \text{ mcg}}{1000} = 0.713 \text{ mg } answer$$

Nomogram for determination of body surface area from height and weight

Height	Body surface area	Weight

Example:

Using the nomogram: A patient's weight is 80 Kg and height is 6'6". The physician orders his chemotherapy treatment as 6.5 mg/m^2 once daily for five days. How many mg of drug will the patient receive in one day?

From the nomogram BSA = 2.30m^2

Set up a ratio and proportion

$$\frac{6.5\ mg}{1m^2} = \frac{X}{2.30\ m^2} \rightarrow \frac{X \times \cancel{1m^2}}{\cancel{1m^2}} = \frac{6.5\ mg \times 2.30\ \cancel{m^2}}{1\cancel{m^2}}$$

→ X = 14.95 mg *answer*

From the formula of Du Bois and Du Bois, *Arch. inture. Med.*, 17, 863 (1916): S = W$^{8.466}$ × H$^{8.766}$ × 71.84, or log S = log W × 0.425 + log H × 0.725 + 1.8564 (S = body surface in cm^2, W = weight in kg, H = height in cm). From *Scientific Tables*, 7th ed. Basel, J. R. Geighy, p. 537.

PRACTICE PROBLEMS

STUDENT NAME _____

DATE _____ COURSE NUMBER _____

1. A physician orders a bolus dose of doxorubicin for a patient with a BSA of 0.96 m². The drug dose is 75 mg/m². What is the bolus dose in mg?

2. A patient weighs 98 pounds and is 5'1" tall. Using the nomogram, find the patient's BSA. The dose of vincristine ordered by the physician is 10 mg/m² per day. What will be the dose in mg?

3. A patient with a BSA of 1.95 is ordered a dose of doxorubicin of 40 mg/m² two times daily. What will be the daily dose, in mg, for this patient?

4. Using the nomogram, find the BSA for the following patient: Weight is 64 Kg, height is 5'6". The physician orders a dose of vinblastine of 1.6 mg/m² daily for four days. Calculate the number of milligrams received by the patient over the four days.

5. A patient's weight is 70 Kg and height is 155 centimeters. Calculate the dose of fluorouracil, in mg, for the patient if the oncologist orders 400 mg/m² daily.

6.   A patient has a BSA of 1.54. The physician orders a daily dose of 900 mg/m^2 of methotrexate for this patient. What is the daily dose, in ml, if the concentration of methotrexate available is 25 mg/ml?

7.   A physician order is for Adriamycin 25 mg/m^2 daily for four days. The patient has a 2.5 BSA. What is the total amount, in mg, that the patient will receive over the four days?

8.   A patient with 1.8 BSA is to receive mesna 4500 mg/m^2 IV in 1000 ml D$_5$W over 18 hours on day one of treatment. Mesna is available as 1000 mg/ml vials. Calculate how many ml are required for the IV bag.

9.   The physician for a patient, BSA 1.9, orders cisplatin 15 mg/m^2 continuous infusion. Cisplatin is available in 50 ml vials with a concentration of 1 mg/ml. How many ml will be required for this order?

10.   Taxotere is ordered 55 mg per m^2 over one hour. The patient has a BSA of 1.93. Taxotere is available in a concentration of 20 mg/ml. Calculate how many ml are needed for this patient's dose.

11.   A patient weighs 184 pounds and is 72 inches in height. The physician orders doxorubicin 25 mg/m^2 IV push. The doxorubicin is supplied as 50 mg vials reconstituted to 4 mg/ml. How many ml will this patient need for his IV push?

12.   A patient with a BSA of 1.52 is ordered leukovorin 100 mg/m² IV in 100 ml 0.9% sodium chloride solution over one hour. Leukovorin is supplied as 200 mg dry powder that is reconstituted to 10 mg/ml. Calculate how many ml are to be added to the IV bag.

13.   5FU 400 mg/m² as IV push is ordered for a patient—whose height is 60.5 inches and weight is 123.4 pounds. 5FU is available as 50 mg/ml in 10 ml vials. How many ml will the patient require?

14.   Topetecan 1 mg/m² IV over 30 minutes in 50 ml of Normal Saline is ordered for a patient with a BSA of 2.00. Topetecan is supplied as 4 mg/vial reconstituted to 1 mg/ml. How many ml will be added to the IV bag?

15.   A patient with a BSA 1.8 is to receive Cytoxan 4500 mg/m² IV in 1000 ml of 0.9% Sodium Chloride Injection over 12 hours. Cytoxan is supplied as 2 g vials 50 mg/ml after reconstitution. How many ml should the technician add to the IV bag?

16.   A patient with a BSA of 1.52 is to receive etoposide 2000 mg/m² via a syringe pump over two hours. Etoposide is supplied as 525 mg/25 ml vials. How many ml will be needed for this patient?

17.   Bleomycin 10 units/m² IV push is ordered for a patient with a BSA 2.05. Bleomycin is available as 15 units/ml. Calculate how many ml are needed for this patient's dose.

18. A patient, whose weight is 80.5 Kg and height is 63 inches, is to receive dacarbazine 375 mg/m² in 250 ml 5% Dextrose Injection over 30 to 60 minutes. Dacarbazine is available as 200 mg/vial reconstituted to 10 mg/ml. How many ml will be needed to add to the IV bag?

19. Paclitaxel 45 mg/m² in 500 ml Normal Saline is to be given to a patient with BSA 2.1. Paclitaxel is supplied as 6 mg/ml. How many ml should the technician add to the IV bag?

20. A physician orders carboplatin, 360 mg/m² in 250 ml Normal Saline infused over one hour. The patient has a BSA of 2.6. How many ml must the technician add to the IV bag? Carboplatin is available after reconstitution in a concentration of 10 mg/ml.

21. A physician orders a 375 mg/m² dose of Rituxan in 500 mls NS for a patient with a BSA of 1.24 m². Rituxan is available in 10 ml vials in a concentration of 10 mg/ml. How many mls will be added to the IV bag?

22. Cyclophosphamide, after reconstitution, has a concentration of 20 mg/ml. The patient, who weighs 67 Kg and is 155 cm tall, is ordered cyclophosphamide 600 mg/m² in 250 mls NS. How many mls will be added to the bag?

23. Doxorubicin, after reconstitution, is available as a 2 mg/ml solution. The physician orders a syringe for IV push at a dose of 35 mg/m². The patient has a BSA of 1.2 m². How many mls are drawn into the syringe?

24.   A patient is to receive Taxol 175 mg/m². She weighs 90 pounds and is 5'2" tall. The Taxol is available, after reconstitution, in a concentration of 6 mg/ml. How many mls will be added to a 500 ml bag of NS for IV infusion?

25.   An order is received in the pharmacy for 5-FU IV for a patient with a BSA of 1.6 m². The 5-FU solution is available in a 50 mg/ml concentration. The dosage schedule is as follows:

Initial dose: 400 mg/m² for 5 days IV push
How many grams of 5-FU has the patient received for the initial dose?

26.   50 mg of a powdered drug is reconstituted with 10 ml of Sterile Water for Injection (assume no powder volume). A patient is ordered an 85 mg/m² dose of the drug in 250 ml D_5W. The patient's BSA is 0.82 m². How many mls of the reconstituted drug will be added to the IV bag?

27.   A patient weighs 180 pounds and is 6'2" tall. The dose of a drug ordered by his physician is 1.3 mg/m² IV push twice weekly for two weeks. The drug is available in a concentration of 1 mg/ml. How many mls of the ordered drug will the patient receive for each dose?

28.   A patient, weight 125 pounds, height 5'6", is to receive the following chemotherapy regime: 800 mcg/m² twice weekly for 2 weeks. The chemo drug when reconstituted has a concentration of 1 mg/ml. How many mls of the drug will the patient receive for the complete regime?

29. The initial loading dose of a chemo drug is 400 mg/m² infused over
     120 minutes and the maintenance dose is 250 mg/m² infused over
     60 minutes. The drug is available as 12 mg/ml. The patient, BSA
     1.2 m², received a 25 ml dose. Is this an initial or maintenance
     dose?

30. A physician orders bleomycin in a dose of 20 units/m² twice weekly.
     The reconstituted bleomycin has a concentration of 30 units/5 ml. The
     patient has a BSA of 2.5 m². How many mls will the patient need for
     a single dose?

31. An order is received in the pharmacy for methotrexate 40 mg/m².
     Methotrexate is available in a concentration of 2.5 mg/ml. How many
     mls are needed for the dose for the patient (weight 80 Kg, height
     160 cm)?

32. A physician orders mesna 1.33 G/m²/day. The pharmacy has on hand
     mesna 100 mg/ml. The patient has a BSA of 0.8 m². How many mls
     will the patient receive each day?

33. A 155-pound patient (height 5'9") is ordered interferon Alfa-2b IM
     2 million units/m² 3 times a week. The drug is available 10 MU in
     1 ml. How many mls will the patient need per week?

34. In the pharmacy, idarubicin is available as a 1 mg/ml solution for IV use. The patient, with a BSA of 1.5 m² is ordered 12 mg/m²/day for 3 days by slow IV. How many mls will be administered for the total treatment?

35. 20 ml Sterile Water for Injection is added to a 1 G vial of powdered ifosfamide (assume no powder volume). The order for the patient is 700 mg/m² IV push. How many mls of the reconstituted ifosfamide will be drawn into the syringe? The patient has a BSA of 1.1 m².

36. The patient is to receive a rapid bolus dose of Alkeran within the hour. The order is for 16 mg/m². Alkeran is reconstituted to 5 mg/ml. The patient has a BSA of 1.92 m². How many mls of the reconstituted solution will the patient need?

37. Robaxin Injection is available in a 10 ml vial with a concentration of 100 mg/ml. An order is received in the pharmacy for Robaxin Injection 500 mg/m²/dose that may be repeated in 6 hours. The patient weighs 68 pounds and is 4'10" tall. How many mls will the patient need for one dose?

38. A 1G vial of methotrexate when reconstituted with Normal Saline has a concentration of 50 mg/ml. A patient with a BSA of 1.39 m² is ordered 6 G/m² by IV infusion every week. How many mls of the reconstituted solution will the patient receive?

39. A chemo drug is available in the pharmacy as 50 mg capsules. A patient with a BSA of 1.66 m^2 is ordered 60 mg/m^2/day for 14 days. How many capsules will the patient require for this course of treatment?

40. Leukine is to be administered by IV at 250 mcg/m^2/day for 21 days. The standard diluted dose in use is 250 mcg/25 ml NS. How many mls will a patient with a BSA of 2.1 m^2 require each day?

33 Infusion Rates and Drip Rates

PHYSICIANS WRITE ORDERS for the rate at which an IV is infused into a patient. Infusion rates can be expressed as number of milliliters per minute, milliliters per hour, amount of drug per hour, and often as the length of time for a volume to be infused. For example:

- Infuse at 125 ml/hr

- Infuse 1000 ml over 8 hours

- Infuse 10 mg per minute

If the volume of the infusion and the time of the infusion are known, then the rate of infusion can be calculated from the following formula:

$$\frac{Volume}{Time} = Rate$$

Example:

Infuse 1000 ml over 8 hours. What is the rate of infusion in ml/hr?

$$\frac{1000\ ml}{8\ hr} = Rate \rightarrow 125\ ml/hr$$

The time of an infusion can be calculated using the same formula. For example, if the rate of infusion is 100 ml/hr and the volume of the infusion is 1000 ml, how long will this bag last?

$$\frac{1000\ ml}{Time} = 100\ ml/hr \rightarrow Time = \frac{1000\ \cancel{ml}}{100\ \cancel{ml}/hr} \rightarrow 10\ hours$$

Similarly, the volume of an infusion can be calculated using the same formula.

Infusions that are administered to a patient by gravity flow are infused through IV sets that are calibrated in drops per milliliter. The rate of infusion is expressed as drops per minute.

Conversions are made to a flow rate of drops per minute from the infusion rate ordered by physicians.

To convert a flow rate in ml/hr to drops/min, two steps are involved.

Example:

The flow rate of an IV infusion ordered by a physician is 125 ml/hr. The IV set to be used for the infusion is calibrated at 15 drops/ml. Calculate the rate of flow in drops/min.

Convert the flow rate from ml/hr to ml/min. 1 hour = 60 minutes

Set up a ratio and proportion.

$$\frac{125 \text{ ml}}{60 \text{ mins}} = \frac{X}{1 \text{ min}} \quad \rightarrow \quad X \times \frac{\cancel{60 \text{ min}}}{\cancel{60 \text{ min}}} = \frac{125 \text{ ml} \times 1\cancel{\text{min}}}{60 \cancel{\text{min}}}$$

→ X = 2.08 → 2.1 ml/min

Calculate the drops for 2.1 ml/min using the calibration of the IV set → 15 drops/ml.

Set up a ratio and proportion.

$$\frac{15 \text{ drops}}{1 \text{ ml}} = \frac{X}{2.1 \text{ ml}} \quad \rightarrow \quad X \times \frac{\cancel{1\text{ml}}}{\cancel{1\text{ml}}} = \frac{15 \text{ drops} \times 2.1\cancel{\text{ml}}}{1\cancel{\text{ml}}}$$

→ X = 31.5 → 32 drops/min

All conversions from ml/hr to drops/min can be calculated using this two-step method.

Example:

A physician orders 12,500 units of heparin in a 1000 ml bag of 5% Dextrose Injection for a patient. The rate of infusion is 500 units over one hour. What will be the rate of infusion in ml/hour?

Calculate the volume, in milliliters, that will contain 500 units.

Set up a ratio and proportion problem.

$$\frac{12,500 \text{ units}}{1000 \text{ ml}} = \frac{500 \text{ units}}{X} \quad \rightarrow \quad X = \frac{1000 \text{ ml} \times 500 \cancel{\text{units}}}{12,500 \cancel{\text{units}}}$$

→ X = 40 ml

Flow rate = 40 ml/hr *answer*

STUDENT NAME _____

DATE _____ COURSE NUMBER _____

1. If a 1 liter bag of D_5W is run through an IV into a patient's arm over eight hours, what is the rate of infusion in ml/hr?

2. If a 500 ml bag of 0.9% Sodium Chloride Injection is run over eight hours, what is the rate of infusion?

3. If a 1000 ml bag of Normal Saline is run at 100 ml/hr, how long will the bag last?

4. A sterile solution request form is received for a large volume parenteral. The infusion rate is 125 ml/hr. The nurse requests enough 1 liter bags for the next 24 hours. How many bags do you make?

5. If the infusion rate for an IV is 80 ml/hr and it is run for four and a half-hours, how many ml has the patient received?

6. If 1 liter of D_5W is started on a patient at 1400 hours on Tuesday, at what time and day will the next liter be required if the rate is:

   a. 125 ml/hr
      next bag needed at _____ on _____ day

    b. 80 ml/hr
       next bag needed at _____ on _____ day

    c. 200 ml/hr
       next bag needed at _____ on _____ day

    d. 50 cc/hr
       next bag needed at _____ on _____day

7. Potassium chloride 30 mEq is to be given in 1 liter of IV fluid. The infusion rate is 125 ml/hr. How many mEq/hr are being infused?

8. A 50 ml IVPB bag of ampicillin 500 mg in Normal Saline is to be run in over 20 minutes. What is the infusion rate in ml/hr?

9. An order is for heparin IV to infuse at 1000 units per hour. What will be the flow rate in ml/hr for a 500 ml bag of D_5W with 25,000 units of heparin?

10. A patient is on a heparin drip, 12,500 units in 250 ml of 0.45% Sodium Chloride Injection. He is to receive 1500 units per hour. At what rate (ml/hr) should the drug be infused?

11. How many drops per minute will a patient receive if an IV of 1000 ml of 5% Dextrose Injection is run in over eight hours? The drip factor is 15 drops/ml.

12. One hundred micrograms of a drug, dissolved in 240 ml of solution, is to be infused at a rate of 75 mcg/hr. If 1 ml = 15 drops, what should the rate of administration be in drops/min?

13. Calculate the infusion rate in ml/hr for a drip, concentration 5 gm/500 ml. The rate is 25 mcg/Kg/min. The patient weighs 112 Kg.

14. What is the flow rate, in drops/min, for a TPN compounded with 500 ml of $D_{10}W$ and 500 ml 7% Travasol run in over 24 hours? The IV administration set is calibrated to deliver 10 drops/ml.

15. The physician orders 3000 ml of D_5W IV over a 24-hour period. If the IV set is calibrated to deliver 15 drops per ml, how many drops must be administered per minute?

16. How long will it take to complete an IV infusion of 1.5 L of 0.9% Sodium Chloride Injection being administered at 45 drops/minute? The IV set is calibrated to deliver 15 drops per ml.

17.   Ampicillin 500 mg in 50 ml IVPB is to be administered over a period of 15 minutes. The drop factor for the IV administration set is 10 drops/ml. Calculate the rate of flow in drops per minute.

18.   The drop factor for an IV line is set at 30 drops/min. Calculate the rate of infusion in ml/hr. The drop factor is 15 drops/ml.

19.   You have a 500 ml bottle of an 8% drug. The rate of infusion is 5 g/hr. What is the rate of infusion in ml/hr and how long will the bottle last?

20.   What volume of fluid will a patient receive if a large volume parenteral bag is running at 50 ml/hr and is begun at 0800 and discontinued at 1400?

21.   A physician orders an IV to be infused at 30 mg/minute for 24 hours. What is the total gram dose for this patient?

22.   A patient is to receive 2 G of an antibiotic in 250 ml of D_5W/NS over 1 hour. The rate of infusion is 30 mg/minute. How long will it take for the patient to receive the infusion?

23. The rate of infusion of a drug is 45 ml/hr as ordered by the physician. A bag of 1000 ml of D_5W is hung on day 1 at 0400 hours. What time will the next 1000 ml bag be needed?

24. A 50 ml IVPB bag contains 500,000 units of penicillin G. The rate of infusion ordered by the physician is 120 ml/hr. How long will the IVPB take to infuse?

25. An IV is running at 50 ml/hr. The 500 ml bag contains 180 mEq of potassium chloride. How many mEq of potassium chloride is the patient receiving per hour?

26. A physician orders a drug to be infused at 10 mcg/Kg/min. The patient weighs 70 Kg. The total dose the patient is to receive is 21 mg. How long must the IV continue for the patient to receive this dose?

27. A patient order is for 1000 ml to be infused over 75 minutes. What is the rate of infusion in ml/hr?

28. The infusion rate for 50 ml of D_5W containing 3.5 G of an antibiotic is 200 ml/hr. What is the infusion rate in drops/min if the IV set is calibrated at 10 drops/ml?

29. A 500 ml IV bag of Lactated Ringers is to be infused at 100 ml/hr. How many 500 ml bags will be needed for 24 hours?

30. A 250 ml bag of D_5W is to be infused at 40 drops/min. The IV set drop factor is 60 drops/ml. The IV is started at 6 a.m. When will the next bag be needed?

31. The physician orders a 500 mg loading dose of a drug to be administered over 20 minutes by IV infusion. A 50 ml IVPB containing the 500 mg is supplied. At what rate in ml/hr should the IVPB be infused?

32. An order is received to infuse 750 ml of IV fluid every 6 hours. At what rate should the IV pump be set for (in ml/hr)?

33. A patient is receiving 250 ml of D_5W infusing at 33 gtt/min. The IV tubing is calibrated for 10 gtt/ml. What is the infusion time for the bag?

34. An MD orders a continuous infusion at a rate of 3 ml/min. The 1000 ml IV bag contains a 2 G dose of the medication ordered. How many mg of the drug will the patient receive in 20 minutes?

35. 37 units of Regular Insulin is to be administered over 1 hour as a continuous infusion. The insulin is added to a 250 ml bag of 0.9% Sodium Chloride Solution. What infusion rate (gtt/min) should be used if the IV set is calibrated for 10 drops/ml?

36. A medication is ordered by the physician 2 G in 250 mls NS to be administered by continuous IV around the clock for 24 hours. The rate of infusion is 100 ml/hr. If the first bag is started at 0800, how many bags in total will be needed?

37. With reference to question 36, give the times (in military time) that each bag will be started.

38. A continuous infusion is to be administered at a rate of 2 mg/min. 200 mg of the drug is added to 250 ml of Ringers Solution. What is the rate of infusion in ml/hr?

39. A drug is to be administered at 40 mcg in 25 minutes. The patient is receiving 0.12 mg in 1000 ml of D_5W. What is the rate of infusion in ml/hr?

40. A drug is to be administered at 200 ml/hr. The IV set being used is calibrated at 8 drops/ml. What is the drip rate in gtt/min?

34 Dilutions

SOMETIMES IT IS NECESSARY to dilute a concentrated solution before dispensing. You may need to calculate the percent concentration of a final volume. You may need to prepare a certain percent dilution and calculate the amount of diluent to add to an available solution.

In the following examples, note the phrases in italics. It is important to distinguish between solutions that are diluted to a certain volume and solutions that have additional solution added to make a final volume.

Example:

If 500 ml of a 30% solution is *diluted* to 600 ml, what will be the percent strength of the resulting solution?

This problem may be solved in two steps.

1. Calculate how many grams are contained in 500 ml of the 30% solution.

$$\frac{30 \text{ g}}{100 \text{ ml}} = \frac{X}{500 \text{ ml}} \quad \rightarrow \quad X = \frac{30 \text{ g} \times 500 \text{ ml}}{100 \text{ ml}} \quad \rightarrow \quad 150 \text{ g}$$

2. This 150 g is then diluted in 600 ml. To find the percentage strength, calculate how many grams are in 100 ml/ (By definition % is g per 100 ml.)

$$\frac{150 \text{ g}}{600 \text{ ml}} = \frac{X}{100 \text{ ml}} \quad \rightarrow \quad X = \frac{150 \text{ g} \times 100 \text{ ml}}{600 \text{ ml}} \quad \rightarrow \quad 25 \text{ g} \quad \rightarrow \quad 25\% \text{ } answer$$

Example:

200 ml of a diluent is *added* to 350 ml of a 35% solution. What is the final percent concentration of the diluted solution?

1. Calculate how many grams are contained in 350 ml of 35% solution.

$$\frac{35 \text{ g}}{100 \text{ ml}} = \frac{X}{350 \text{ ml}} \quad \rightarrow \quad X = \frac{35 \text{ g} \times 350 \text{ ml}}{100 \text{ ml}} \quad \rightarrow \quad X = 122.5 \text{ g}$$

Note: The final volume is determined by 200 ml + 350 ml = 550 ml.

2: The 122.5 g is then diluted in 550 ml.

$$\frac{122.5 \text{ g}}{550 \text{ ml}} = \frac{X}{100 \text{ ml}} \quad \rightarrow \quad X = \frac{122.5 \text{ g} \times 100 \text{ ml}}{550 \text{ ml}} \quad \rightarrow \quad X = 22.27 \text{ g}$$

→ 22.27% *answer*

Example:

You *mix together* the following volumes of the same drug: (a) 150 ml of 20% solution; (b) 50 ml of 35% solution, and (c) 20 ml of 50% solution. What is the percent concentration of the final solution after mixing?

1. To solve this problem you need to calculate the total grams from each of the three solutions.

   a. $\dfrac{20 \text{ g}}{100 \text{ ml}} = \dfrac{X}{150 \text{ ml}}$ ➜ $X = \dfrac{20 \text{ g} \times 150 \text{ ml}}{100 \text{ ml}}$ ➜ $X = 30 \text{ g}$

   b. $\dfrac{35 \text{ g}}{100 \text{ ml}} = \dfrac{X}{50 \text{ ml}}$ ➜ $X = \dfrac{35 \text{ g} \times 50 \text{ ml}}{100 \text{ ml}}$ ➜ $X = 17.5 \text{ g}$

   c. $\dfrac{50 \text{ g}}{100 \text{ ml}} = \dfrac{X}{20 \text{ ml}}$ ➜ $X = \dfrac{50 \text{ g} \times 20 \text{ ml}}{100 \text{ ml}}$ ➜ $X = 10 \text{ g}$

Total 57.5 g.

2. The 57.5g is then diluted in the total volume of the three solutions.

   150 ml + 50 ml + 20 ml = 220 ml

   $\dfrac{57.5 \text{ g}}{220 \text{ ml}} = \dfrac{X}{100 \text{ ml}}$ ➜ $X = \dfrac{57.5 \text{ g} \times 100 \text{ ml}}{220 \text{ ml}}$ ➜ $X = 26.14 \text{ g}$

   ➜ 26.14% *answer*

Example:

You are to prepare as much 40% dextrose solution as you can from 200 ml of 70% dextrose solution. How many mls of water do you need to add to the 70% dextrose solution?

1. Calculate how many grams of dextrose is contained in the 200 ml of 70% dextrose solution.

   $\dfrac{70 \text{ g}}{100 \text{ ml}} = \dfrac{X}{200 \text{ ml}}$ ➜ $X = \dfrac{70 \text{ g} \times 200 \text{ ml}}{100 \text{ ml}}$ ➜ $X = 140 \text{ g}$

2. 140 g is available to prepare 40% dextrose solution. Calculate how many mls will be compounded.

   $\dfrac{40 \text{ g}}{100 \text{ ml}} = \dfrac{140 \text{ g}}{X}$ ➜ $X = \dfrac{140 \text{ g} \times 100 \text{ ml}}{40 \text{ g}}$

   ➜ X = 350 ml final solution

3. To find the volume of water required:

   Final volume – volume of 70% dextrose solution

   350 ml – 200 ml = 150 ml water *answer*

STUDENT NAME _____

DATE _____ COURSE NUMBER _____

1. You have 200 ml of a 30% solution. You dilute the solution to 600 ml. What is the percent strength of the final solution?

2. What is the percentage strength of a solution that is made by adding 200 ml of purified water to 600 ml of a 25% solution?

3. You dilute 50 ml of an 8% solution to 500 ml. What is the percentage strength of the resulting solution?

4. A technician has been given 100 ml of a 10% acetic acid solution. The pharmacist asked the technician to dilute the solution to 500 ml with sterile water, and then to label the solution. What % should appear on the label?

5. A 20% solution has been diluted to 400 ml and is now a 5% solution. What was the beginning volume of the 20% solution?

6. You dilute 75 ml of a 30% solution to 500 ml. What is the percentage strength of the final solution prepared?

7. A technician has 50 ml of a 0.5% gentian violet solution on hand. What will be the final percentage strength if she dilutes this solution to 125 ml with purified water?

8. If 2 ml of a 1:200 solution are to be mixed with water to make a final concentration of 1:1000, how much water is needed?

9. You have on hand 200 g of a 40% ointment. This mixture is to be diluted to 320 g with a suitable base. What is the % strength of the resulting ointment?

10. You are preparing a TPN with 500 ml of 7.5% Travasol and 500 ml of 50% Dextrose Injection. What is the final percent concentration of the Travasol and the dextrose in this TPN?

11. A technician is to compound a TPN with 500 ml of 10% Travasol, 250 mls of 70% Dextrose Injection and 350 mls of sterile water. What is the final concentration of the Travasol and the dextrose in the TPN?

12.   You have 4 fluid oz. of a 50% solution and you add 500 ml to this solution. What is the percentage strength of the final solution?

13.   You have 300 ml of a 20% solution of a drug and 400 ml of 5% solution of the same drug. You mix them together. What is the percentage strength of the final solution?

14.   If you mix 100 ml of a 1:100 solution with 350 ml of a 1:200 solution, what is the percentage strength of the final solution? What is the ratio strength of the final solution?

15.   If 14 G of petrolatum are added to 25 G of 0.2% hydrocortisone ointment, what will be the final % concentration of hydrocortisone?

16.   What is the final percentage strength of a solution when 300 ml of 95%, 1000 ml of 70%, and 200 ml of 50% solutions are mixed together?

17.   10 cc of a 50% solution is diluted to 100 cc. What is the % concentration of the diluted solution?

18.   A technician mixes 80 ml of a 5% solution with 10 ml of water. What is the final percentage strength of the solution prepared?

19.   A TPN is composed of 300 ml of 7.5% Travasol and 250 ml of 10% dextrose. What is the final percentage strength of the Travasol and the dextrose in the prepared TPN?

20.   You have on hand 50 ml of 80% dextrose solution and you need to make as much 35% dextrose solution as possible. How much water will you need to add to the 50 ml of 80% dextrose solution?

21.   If 50 ml of a 12% solution is diluted to 120 mls, what is the percentage strength of the new solution?

22.   On hand in the pharmacy is 500 ml of a 16% solution. The technician is asked to dilute this stock solution to obtain a 5% solution. How many mls of distilled water will be required?

23.   How many mls of an 8% Gentian Violet Solution are required to prepare 120 mls of a 1:400 w/v solution?

24. An order is for 60 G of a 3% ointment. On hand is 100 G of a 10% ointment. The 10% ointment must be diluted with petrolatum. How many grams of each ingredient must be used?

25. In the pharmacy is 500 mls of a 75% stock solution. If the technician adds 300 mls to the stock solution, what percentage strength solution is obtained?

26. In the pharmacy are three different percentage strength stock solutions of the same drug. If these are all mixed together, how many mls and what percentage strength solution will result?

120 mls of 75%
54 mls of 10%
20 mls of 8%

27. A 1:1000 w/v solution is required by a patient. On hand in the pharmacy is 20 mls of a 1:250 w/v solution. How many mls of the 1:1000 w/v solution can be made from the stock solution?

28. You mix 500 mls of 7.5% Travasol and 500 mls of 60% dextrose solution and 300 mls of Sterile Water for Injection. What are the percentage strengths of the Travasol and dextrose in the mixed solution?

29. If 200 mls of Sterile Water for Injection is added to 85 mls of an 80% stock solution, what is the percentage strength of the resulting solution?

30. If 700 mls of Sterile Water for Injection is added to 10 mls of a 10% stock solution, what is the ratio strength of the resulting solution?

31. 20 mls of a 1:1000 w/v stock solution is diluted to 200 mls with Sterile Water for Injection. What is the ratio strength of the diluted solution?

32. An order is received for 90 G of a 0.2% ointment. Available in the pharmacy is a 2.5% ointment which can be diluted with petrolatum. How many grams of the 2.5% ointment and how many grams of the petrolatum will be needed?

33. A physician orders 75 mls of a solution that contains 20 G of the required drug. The stock solution in the pharmacy is a 33% solution. How many mls of the stock solution should be diluted with purified water to obtain the strength of the solution ordered by the physician?

34. A technician is asked to prepare a 42% solution. In stock in the pharmacy is 350 mls of a 55% solution. How many mls can the technician prepare if she uses all the stock solution?

35. The total volume of the additives for a TPN is 125 mls. The TPN also contains 500 mls of 7.5% Travasol with lytes and 500 mls of 45% dextrose solution. What is the final % concentration of the Travasol and dextrose when the TPN is completed?

36. A 1:5000 w/v solution is required to fill an order. On hand in the pharmacy is a 1:200 w/v solution. If the order is for 300 mls, how many mls of the stock solution will be needed?

37. A physician orders a liter of half strength Dakin's Solution. On hand in the pharmacy is full strength Dakin's Solution (0.5% sodium hypochlorite solution). How many mls of the stock solution are needed?

38. Available in the pharmacy is 236 mls of a 10% Povidone-Iodine wash concentrate. The physician orders a diluted wash. If 240 ml of 1% Povidone-Iodine wash is ordered, how many mls of the 10% will be needed?

39.   250 mls of a 26.75% solution must be diluted to an 18% solution before administration. How many mls of water must be added?

40.   400 ml of SWFI is added to 1 liter of normal saline solution. What is the percentage strength of the resulting solution?

35 Alligations

IF A CERTAIN PERCENTAGE STRENGTH SOLUTION is needed but not available, a technician can prepare it by mixing together a stronger percentage strength solution and a weaker percentage strength solution in appropriate proportions to achieve the desired strength.

All concentrations must be in a percentage form and the strength of the desired solution must lie between the stronger and weaker solutions available. If the concentration is not expressed in the percentage form, it must be converted to the percentage form. For example, a solution strength expressed as 1:200 must be converted to a percentage.

$$\rightarrow \frac{1}{200} \times 100 = 0.5\%$$

These types of calculations are known as alligations, and they are set up using a layout similar to a tic-tac-toe board.

Higher % Strength Solution ↘		Number of Parts of Higher % Solution
minus	Required % Strength Solution ↗ ↘	
Lower % Strength Solution	minus	Number of Parts of Lower % Solution

- The higher % strength is always placed in the upper left box.

- The lower % strength is always placed in the lower left box.

- The required % strength is always placed in the center box.

- The higher % strength minus the required % strength equals the number of parts of lower % strength solution needed.

- The required % strength minus the lower % strength equals the number of parts of higher % strength solution needed.

- The *total parts* are equal to the sum of the higher % and lower % parts.

- The volume of higher % strength solution needed is determined by dividing the number of parts of higher % strength solution by the total parts and then multiplying by the final volume required.

- Similarly, the volume of lower % strength solution needed is determined by dividing the number of parts of lower % strength solution by the total parts and then multiplying by the final volume required.

Example:

You receive an order for 500 ml of 40% dextrose solution. On hand are stock solutions of 60% dextrose and 25% dextrose. How many ml of each of the stock solutions will you need to prepare this order?

Set up a tic-tac-toe layout.

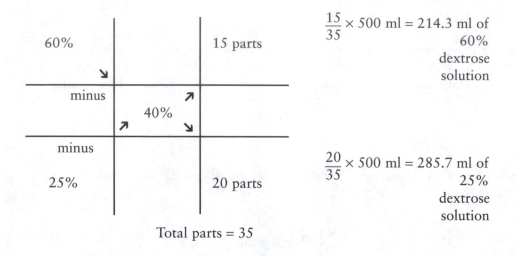

$\dfrac{15}{35} \times 500$ ml = 214.3 ml of 60% dextrose solution

$\dfrac{20}{35} \times 500$ ml = 285.7 ml of 25% dextrose solution

The sum of the volumes for the higher and lower % strengths must equal the final volume.

This method of calculation can also be used when diluting a solution with water. Water is given the value of 0% and is always placed in the lower left box of the tic-tac-toe layout.

Example:

A technician is asked to prepare 350 ml of a 22% boric acid solution from a 50% boric acid solution and purified water. How many ml of 50% solution and water will be needed?

Set up a tic-tac-toe layout.

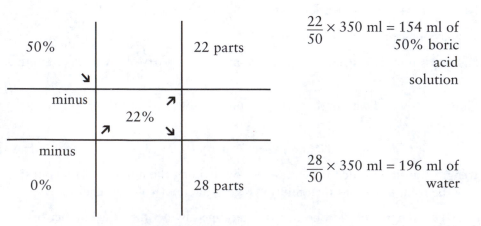

$\dfrac{22}{50} \times 350$ ml = 154 ml of 50% boric acid solution

$\dfrac{28}{50} \times 350$ ml = 196 ml of water

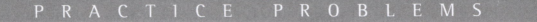

PRACTICE PROBLEMS

STUDENT NAME_____

DATE _____ COURSE NUMBER _____

1. Calculate how many ml of 50% dextrose solution and how many ml of water are needed to prepare 4.5 L of a 1% solution.

2. How many ml of a 50% solution and how many ml of a 5% solution are needed to prepare 4 liters of a 10% solution?

3. How many ml of a 15% solution of sodium chloride and ml of water should be used to prepare 1 liter of a 0.9% solution of sodium chloride?

4. How many ml of each of a 20% stock solution and a 30% stock solution will a technician need to make 500 mls of a 28% solution?

5. How many grams of 10% boric acid ointment should be mixed with petrolatum (0%) to prepare 700 G of a 5% boric acid ointment?

6. You have on hand 10% and 3% ammoniated mercury ointment. You need to prepare 450 g of a 5% ointment. How many grams of each of the 10% and the 3% ointment will you need?

7. A technician is to prepare 2.5 liters of a 1:20 solution from a 30% solution and water. How many ml of the 30% solution and water are needed?

8. A TPN order requires 500 ml of $D_{30}W$. You find that you do not have any $D_{30}W$ in stock, you only have $D_{40}W$ and sterile water. How many ml of $D_{40}W$ and sterile water will you need to complete this order?

9. A hospital clinic requests 2 pounds of 2% hydrocortisone ointment. How many grams of 5% hydrocortisone ointment would be diluted with white petrolatum (0%) to prepare this order?

10. How many ml of a 1:400 stock solution and purified water should be used to prepare 4 liters of a 1:2000 solution?

11. You receive an order for 200 ml of potassium permanganate 1:5000 solution. You have in the pharmacy a 2% potassium permanganate stock solution. How many ml of the stock solution and purified water will you need to compound this prescription?

12. How many ml of a 16% stock solution are needed to compound 400 ml of a 1:2500 solution?

13. Calculate how many ml of a 1:2 solution and ml of water are needed to prepare 50 ml of a 15% solution.

14.   A technician has on hand 70% dextrose stock solution and 40% dextrose stock solution. She is to prepare 1000 ml of 45% dextrose solution. How many ml of each of the stock solutions will she need?

15.   You are to prepare 350 ml of a 1:50 solution from 1:10 and 1:1000 stock solutions. How many ml of each of the stock solutions do you need?

16.   Calculate how many ml of a 30% stock solution and ml of a 85% stock solution are needed to prepare 3 liters of 60% solution.

17.   A physician orders 250 g of a 5% ointment. On hand in the pharmacy are 2% and 10% stock ointments. How many grams of each of the stock ointments are needed to prepare the order?

18.   An order calls for 16 fl. oz. of a 20% solution. On hand are stock solutions of 80% and 8%. How many ml of each of the stock solutions are needed to fill the order?

19.   A technician is asked to prepare a prescription for 10 fl. oz. of a 35% solution. In stock is a 50% solution. How many ml of the 50% stock solution and how many ml of purified water are needed to prepare the prescription?

20.   A prescription is written for 4 fl. oz. of a 7.5% solution. How many fl. oz. each of a 10% stock solution and purified water will be needed to compound this prescription?

21.   In the pharmacy are two stock solutions 50% and 20%. How many mls of each solution will be needed to prepare 800 mls of a 33% solution?

22.   Stock solutions of 27% and 31% are available in the pharmacy. How many mls of each stock solution are needed to prepare 2 liters of a 29% solution?

23.   Two very dilute stock solutions are available to prepare 60 mls of a 1:1000 w/v solution. The two stock solutions are 1:200 w/v and 1:2000 w/v. How many mls of each will be required?

24.   Hydrogen peroxide stock solution is available in a 3.5% strength. How many mls of stock solution and water will be needed to prepare 120 mls of a 2.5% solution?

25.   The technician is asked to prepare 2.5 L of D_5W from a 45% dextrose solution and SWFI. How many mls of each will be needed?

26.   An order is received for 60 G of a 1% ointment. Available in the pharmacy is 100 G of 2.5% ointment. How many grams of the 2.5% ointment and petrolatum (used for dilution of the ointment) will be required?

27.   A pint of 4% solution is ordered. On hand are 1% and 6% stock solutions. How many fluid ounces of each will be needed to fill the prescription?

28. An order is received for 2 quarts of a 14% solution. Purified water and a 20% solution are to be used for the preparation. How many fluid ounces of each are needed?

29. A technician is to prepare 500 mls of a 1:400 w/v solution from a 1% solution and purified water. How many mls of each will be needed?

30. From two stock solutions, 18% and 42%, you are to prepare 1.5 L of a 34% solution. How many mls of each of the stock solutions do you need?

31. An order for 60 mls of a 1% topical liquid is to be prepared from a 5% solution and purified water. How many mls of each are needed?

32. An order for 6 liters of 0.9% sodium chloride solution is to be prepared from 23.4% concentrated NaCl solution and Sterile Water for Injection. How many mls of each will be used?

33. Silver Nitrate Topical Solution is available in 25% and 50% stock solutions. An order is received for 30 mls of 30% solution. How many mls of each of the stock solutions will be needed?

34. An order is received for 50 mls of 7.2% solution to be prepared from 4.2% and 8.4% stock solutions. How many mls of each of the stock solutions will be needed?

35. On hand in the pharmacy are two stock solutions, 0.75% and 3%. A prescription is for 15 mls of a 1.5% solution. How many mls of the two stock solutions are required?

36. A technician is to prepare 250 mls of a 40% solution from a 60% stock solution and purified water. How many mls of each are needed?

37. An order reads 30 mls of 0.6% solution. Available in the pharmacy are two stock solutions, 0.4% and 5%. How many mls of each stock solution will be used to fill the order?

38. The pharmacy has run out of 500 ml bags of 1/2 NS. The technician is to use 0.9% sodium chloride solution and Sterile Water for Injection to make a 500 ml bag of 1/2 NS. How many mls of NS and SWFI will she need?

39. The technician is to prepare 800 G of a 3% ointment. In the pharmacy is a 10% ointment and petrolatum. How many grams of the stock ointment and petrolatum will he or she weigh out?

40. A liter of 1/3 NS is to be prepared from 23.4% concentrated sodium chloride solution and Sterile Water for Injection. How many mls of each are to be used?

36 Parenteral Nutrition Calculations

PARENTERAL NUTRITION SOLUTIONS (also known as hyperalimentation solutions) are a means of providing nutrition to patients via IV, either to replace or maintain essential nutrients.

There are two main types of parenteral nutrition solutions:

- Total Parenteral Nutrition (TPN): These solutions provide all nutrients for a patient.

- Partial Parenteral Nutrition (PPN): These solutions provide some nutrients parenterally combined with other types of feeding such as enteral and/or oral feeding.

Some indications for parenteral nutrition include: gastrointestinal disease, malnutrition, major organ failure, major surgery, and cancer.

A TPN consists of a base solution and additives.

Base Solution

1. Carbohydrates obtained from high concentration dextrose solutions 10% to 70%.

2. Proteins obtained from amino acids solutions 3.5% to 15% (brand names such as Travasol and Aminosyn).

3. Essential fatty acids from fat emulsions 10% and 20%.

Note: The fat emulsion is not always admixed into the TPN. If it is included, the TPN is known as a 3-in-1 TPN. Fat emulsions may be administered to the patient as a separate infusion.

Additives

1. Electrolytes such as sodium chloride, potassium chloride, calcium gluconate, magnesium sulfate, sodium acetate, and potassium phosphates. Electrolytes are prescribed according to patient needs as determined from blood levels.

   Care must be taken when adding a calcium and a phosphate to a TPN. In certain concentrations, these electrolytes are incompatible and a precipitate will form. To minimize this problem, the phosphate is added first to the TPN to allow for dilution of the phosphate and the calcium is added last after all other additives.

2. Vitamins

3. Trace elements

4. Insulin

5. Other additives as prescribed

Typically a TPN will have 6 to 10 additives mixed with the base solution. There is, therefore, a large number of calculations to be performed so great care must be taken and a check by a second person is desirable.

Physicians may prescribe TPNs in a variety of ways:

- Standard formulation: This is a TPN formula developed by the institution, and physicians use this if appropriate for their patient's needs.

- Patient specific: Amino acids, dextrose, and lipids are ordered as grams, and/or grams per kilogram of body weight; electrolytes are ordered as milliequivalents (mEq) or millimoles (mM), and/or mEq or mM per kilogram of body weight.

Calculations for TPN additives may be performed using the ratio and proportion method described earlier in this text.

Example:

Dose required is KCl 30 mEq. The concentration available is 2 mEq/ml.

Set up a ratio and proportion:

$$\frac{2\text{mEq}}{1\text{ ml}} = \frac{30\text{ mEq}}{X} \; \rightarrow \; \frac{X \times \cancel{2\text{mEq}}}{\cancel{2\text{mEq}}} = \frac{1\text{ ml} \times 30\cancel{\text{mEq}}}{2\cancel{\text{mEq}}}$$

$\rightarrow$ X = 15 ml *answer*

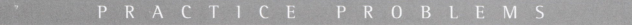

PRACTICE PROBLEMS

STUDENT NAME_____

DATE _____ COURSE NUMBER _____

For all the TPN calculations in this section, use the following concentrations:

Potassium chloride	2 mEq/ml	
Sodium chloride	14.6%	2.5 mEq/ml
Calcium gluconate	10%	4.65 mEq/10ml
Magnesium sulfate	50%	40.6 mEq/10ml
Sodium acetate	2 mEq/ml	
Sodium phosphate	45 mM/15 ml	60 mEq/15 ml
Potassium acetate	19.6%	2 mEq/ml
Potassium phosphate	15 mM/5 ml	4.4 mEq/ml
Humulin R insulin	100 units/ml	
Vitamin C	250 mg/2 ml	

For the following TPN formulas, No. 1 through No. 8, calculate the ml required for each additive.

Example

TPN No. 1: sodium chloride ordered is 25 mEq.

Concentration of sodium chloride available = 2.5 mEq/ml. (Remember, you must use the same units.)

Set up a ratio and proportion:

$$\frac{2.5 \text{ mEq}}{1 \text{ ml}} = \frac{25 \text{ mEq}}{X} \quad \rightarrow \quad \frac{X \times 2.5 \text{ mEq}}{2.5 \text{ mEq}} = \frac{1 \text{ ml} \times 25 \text{ mEq}}{2.5 \text{ mEq}}$$

➔ X = 10 ml *answer*

BASE SOLUTIONS	No. 1	No. 2	No. 3	No. 4
Travasol 7.5 % with lytes	500 ml		500 ml	500 ml
Travasol 10 % without lytes		500 ml		
Dextrose 70 %	500 ml	350 ml	300 ml	500 ml
Sterile Water for Injection		250 ml	200 ml	
Rate ml/hr	60 ml/hr	60 ml/hr	60 ml/hr	60 ml/hr
ADDITIVES				
Sodium chloride	25 mEq	12 mEq	15 mEq	20 mEq
Potassium chloride	30 mEq	20 mEq	10 mEq	14 mEq
Magnesium sulfate	12 mEq	20 mEq	500 mg	2 G
Potassium phosphates	22 mEq	9 mM	12 mM	17.6 mEq
Calcium gluconate	56 mEq	1 G	1.5 G	24 mEq
MVI-12 10ml/vial	10 ml	10 ml	10 ml	10 ml
Trace elements	5 ml	5 ml	5 ml	5 ml
Vitamin C	125 mg	500 mg	625 mg	750 mg
Humulin R insulin	55 units	60 units	80 units	95 units
Folic acid (5mg/ml)	2.5 mg	5 mg	6.25 mg	3.75 mg
Sodium acetate	40 mEq	35 mEq	10 mEq	14 mEq
Potassium acetate	14 mEq	20 mEq	25 mEq	8 mEq
Sodium phosphates	4 mEq	20 mEq	8 mEq	12 mM

5. A patient is ordered the following TPN. Calculate the milliliters needed for each additive. (Use the concentrations provided previously.)

Base Solutions:	7.5% Travasol	500 mls
	60% Dextrose solution	500 mls

Additives:	Potassium chloride	84 mEq
	Sodium chloride	60 mEq
	Magnesium sulfate	8 mEq
	Trace elements	5 mls
	Sodium acetate	20 mEq
	Humulin R insulin	54 units
	Calcium gluconate	2.5 G

What are the final % concentrations of Travasol and dextrose in the TPN?

6. **The following TPN is ordered for a patient whose weight is 20 Kg. Calculate the milliliters needed for each additive.**

Base Solutions:	5% Travasol	250 mls
	20% Dextrose solution	150 mls
Additives:	Sodium chloride	3 mEq/Kg
	Potassium chloride	2.5 mEq/Kg
	Calcium gluconate	1.5 mEq/Kg
	Magnesium sulfate	0.5 mEq/Kg
	Potassium phosphate	1 mMol/Kg

What are the % concentrations of the Travasol and the dextrose in the completed TPN?

7. **Calculate the milliliters needed for each additive in the following TPN.**

Base Solutions:	10% Travasol	1000 mls
	50% Dextrose solution	1000 mls
	Sterile Water for Injection	500 mls
Additives:	Potassium chloride	120 mEq
	Sodium chloride	86 mEq
	Magnesium sulfate	24 mEq
	Calcium gluconate	9 mEq
	Trace elements	5 mls
	MVI	10 mls
	Potassium phosphate	40 mMol
	Humulin R insulin	68 units

Calculate the final % strengths of the base solutions in the compounded TPN.

8. **A TPN is to be compounded with the following medications. Calculate the milliliters required for each additive.**

Base Solutions:	8.5% Aminosyn	550 mls
	60% Dextrose solution	500 mls

Additives:	Potassium chloride	140 mEq
	Sodium chloride	105 mEq
	Magnesium sulfate	1 G
	Calcium gluconate	2 G
	Potassium phosphate	13.2 mEq
	Vitamin C	750 mg

What are the final % concentrations of the Aminosyn and the dextrose in the TPN?

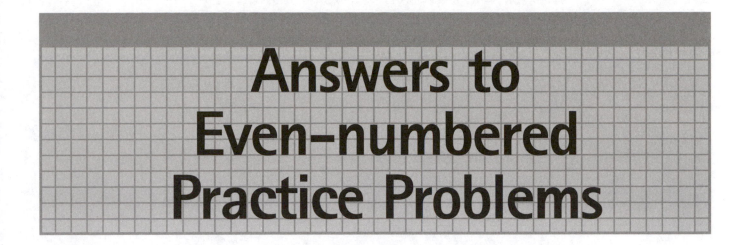

Answers to Even-numbered Practice Problems

1 Numeral Systems Used in Pharmacy

2. 90
4. 32
6. 22
8. 4
10. 19
12. 109
14. 8
16. 34
18. 28
20. 29
22. XX
24. XL
26. XV
28. CC
30. M
32. VII
34. XVI
36. XXXVI
38. LVII
40. CM

2 Numerators, Denominators, and Reciprocals of Fractions

2. 0.25
4. 0.4
6. 0.125
8. 0.05
10. 0.001
12. 0.75
14. 0.33
16. 0.143
18. 0.833
20. 0.278
22. 0.273
24. 0.091
26. 0.163
28. 0.206
30. 0.277
32. 4/1 = 4
34. 5/2 = 2 1/2
36. 8/1 = 8
38. 20/1 = 20
40. 1,000/1 = 1,000
42. 4/3

44. 3/1 = 3
46. 7/1 = 7
48. 6/5
50. 18/5
52. 23/3 = 7 2/3
54. 12/5 = 2 2/5
56. 48/7 = 6 6/7
58. 23/9 = 2 5/9
60. 83/23 = 3 14/23

3 Reducing Fractions to Lowest Terms

2. 1/4
4. 1/8
6. 1/3
8. 1/22
10. 13/15
12. 4/5
14. 1/5
16. 3/4
18. 2/5
20. 7/18
22. 0
24. 2/5

26. 5/6

28. 2/3

30. 2/3

32. 6/25

34. 2/3

36. 12/35

38. 2/9

40. 2/17

42. 1/4

44. 1/10

46. 1/9

48. 1/2

50. 1/6

52. 2/9

54. 2/5

56. 1/2

58. 7/15

60. 3/7

4   Adding and Subtracting Fractions

2. 4/8 = 1/2

4. 2/8 = 1/4

6. 4/8 = 1/2

8. 9/25

10. 5/8

12. 4/5

14. 10/15 = 2/3

16. 11/10

18. 5/12

20. 5 703/1000

22. 1/6

24. 1/14

26. 4/20 = 1/5

28. 343/432

30. 409/1000

32. 14/8 = 1 3/4

34. 17/18

36. 26/18 = 1 4/9

38. 41/38 = 1 3/38

40. 23/20 = 1 3/20

42. 17/24

44. 187/198

46. 27/24 = 1 1/4

48. 25/36

50. 15/152

5   Multiplying and Dividing Fractions

2. 3/64

4. 15/64

6. 21/64

8. 3/20

10. 8/21

12. 2/27

14. 4/125

16. 7/32

18. 7/64

20. 10

22. 48/455

24. 0

26. 3/420 = 1/140

28. 3/384 = 1/128

30. 30/504 = 5/84

32. 1/480

34. 15/384 = 5/128

36. 1

38. 2

40. 1/3

42. 5/3 = 1 2/3

44. 2/3

46. 5/8

48. 4/3 = 1 1/3

50. 1/15

52. 49/25

54. 0

56. 1/6

58. 125

60. 100

62. 25

64. 32

66. 200

68. 300

70. 5,000

6   Writing Fractions in Decimal Form

2. 0.033

4. 35.153

6. 0.86

8. 0.3

10. 0.17

12. 60.028

14. 850.0036

16. ninety-three hundredths

18. thirty-two and fifty-eight hundredths

20. thirty-five and seventy-eight thousandths

22. eighteen and one hundred two thousandths

24. six hundred seven and six hundred seven thousandths

26. 63/100

28. 88/100

30. 2/10

32. 47/100

34. 41/100

36. 1 35/100

38. 4 53/100

40. 10 353/1000

42. 31 451/1000

44. 51 118/1000

7 Rounding Decimals and Significant Figures

2. 6.99

4. 235,121.35

6. 2.34

8. 3.23

10. 136.57

12. 7.6

14. 37.7

16. 0.0

18. 44.4

20. 0.2

22. 56

24. 1

26. 1

28. 3

30. 3

32. 54

34. 325

36. 480

38. 1,001

40. 346

42. 3

44. 2

8 Adding and Subtracting Decimal Numbers

2. 11.5

4. 45.083

6. 4.6926

8. 83.315

10. 481.25

12. 25.4

14. 317.8

16. 32.8

18. 36.168

20. 245.9853

22. 230.4465

24. 22,381.15

26. 1.44

28. 15.89

30. 64.947

32. 4.7974

34. 2.9434

36. 1.68

38. 1.01

40. 0.2

42. 11.1

44. 109.9

46. 349.122

48. 5,157.9095

50. 12.1220875

9 Multiplying Decimal Numbers

2. 0.24

4. 0.09

6. 38.4

8. 0.9

10. 0.009

12. 0.073

14. 0.0225

16. 0.0568

18. 0.0025

20. 223.3

22. 14.52

24. 7.938402

26. 332.212

28. 5.024

30. 54.945

32. 1,784.2176

34. 14,663

36. 0.04222

38. 1

40. 779.2876

42. 8.175

44. 2.626745

46. 4.03293

10 Using Ratios and Proportions or Dimensional Analysis to Solve Pharmacy Calculations

2. 6

4. 2

6. 12

8. 1

10. 3

12. 5

14. 6

16. 60

18. 1,000

20. 14

22. 20

24. 90

26. 68

28. 20

30. 6

32. 56

34. 102

36. 63

38. 12

40. 21

11 Percents

2. 0.24

4. 0.505

6. 0.47

8. 0.325

10. 0.8332

12. 0.185

14. 0.0025

16. 24.44%

18. 50%

20. 75%

22. 9%

24. 80%

26. 52%

28. 65%

30. 3.5%

32. 0.4%

34. 175%

36. 150

38. 3

40. 3

42. 90

44. 5.5

46. 2.5

48. 20

50. 280

52. 20%

54. 75%

56. 85%

58. 42.9%

60. 60%

62. 80%

64. 88.9%

66. 10

68. 4.8

70. 12

72. 50

74. 27

12 Exponents and Scientific Notation

2. 1

4. 1,000

6. 46,656

8. 100,000

10. 3,125

12. 64

14. 49

16. 100

18. 16,384

20. 216

22. 4.56×10 EE 2

24. 78.322×10 EE 3

26. 1.567334×10 EE 6

28. 1.25×10 EE -1

30. 8×10 EE 0

32. 1×10 EE 3

34. 1.5×10 EE 1

36. 6.1×10 EE 3

38. 5.03×10 EE 2

40. 1×10 EE 6

13 Converting Household and Metric Measurements

2. 15

4. 227

6. 2.5

8. 11,355

10. 59.2

12. 1,419

14. 1/5

16. 3

18. 6

20. 4

22. 9

24. 45

26. 2.27

28. 946

30. 1.98

32. 1

34. 1

36. 8.75

38. 6

40. 3

42. 1 teaspoonful

44. 1/4 teaspoonful

14 Converting Apothecary and Metric Measurements

2. 32.4

4. 15

6. 1.852 (rounds to 2)

8. 4

10. 118.4 (rounds to 120)

12. 10

14. 186

16. 25

18. 372

20. 12

22. 1/2

24. 24

26. 1.5

28. 1.25

30. 248

32. 129.6

34. 3,086.4

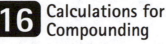 **15 Converting Between the Different Temperature Scales**

2. 59 degrees Fahrenheit

4. 113 degrees Fahrenheit

6. 68 degrees Fahrenheit

8. 86 degrees Fahrenheit

10. 122 degrees Fahrenheit

12. 90 degrees Fahrenheit

14. 36 degrees Fahrenheit

16. 23 degrees Fahrenheit

18. 45 degrees Fahrenheit

20. 64 degrees Fahrenheit

22. 21 degrees Celsius

24. −9 degrees Celsius

26. 24 degrees Celsius

28. −4 degrees Celsius

30. 38 degrees Celsius

32. −11 Celsius

34. 3 Celsius

36. 14 Celsius

38. 26 Celsius

40. 32 Celsius

16 Calculations for Compounding

2. 15 grams, 1.25%

4. 30 tablets

6. 3 grams

8. 25 tablets

10. 10 capsules

12. 10 ml

14. 7

16. 15

18. 1

20. 6

22. 12

24. 7

26. 3

28. 10

30. 0.2 ml

17 Calculations for Days Supply

2. 14

4. 10

6. 15

8. 5

10. 10

12. 15–30 (explanation: 1–2 ml per application depending on the area treated)

14. 15

16. 28

18. 2

20. 3 (explanation: for ophthalmic ointments estimate is 100 mg per eye per application)

22. 3

24. 7 (explanation: see package, package insert, or reference book for packaging information)

26. 6

28. 84

30. 10

32. 30

34. 10

36. 15

38. 40

40. 30

42. 30

44. 10

46. 7

48. 10

18 Adjusting Refills for Short-filled Prescriptions

2. 5 boxes + 5 refills

4. 68 + 2 refills of 68 (leaving a partial refill of 36)

6. 1 + 7 refills

8. 1 + 1 refill

10. 34 + 6 refills (leaving a partial refill of 2)

12. 240, 1, 0

14. 136, 1, 128

16. 1 pt., 1, 0

18. 68, 3, 28

20. 34, 10, 26

22. 34, 0, 16

24. 102, 1, 36

26. 34, 4, 30

28. 68, 3, 28

30. 102, 4, 90

19 Calculations for Dispensing Fees, Co-pays, Difference Pricing

2. $15.66 ($7.00 + ($12.74 – $4.08))

4. $25.11 ((0.2*$12.08) + ($34.77 – $12.08))

6. $18

8. $26.00

10. $97

12. $74.70

14. $40.10

16. $54.50

18. $44.50

20. $69.90

22. $117.70

24. $101.50

20 Calculations for Billing Compounds

2. $17.64

4. $24.20

6. $24.32

8. $34.32

10. $51.14

12. $21.22

14. $16.77

16. $21.70

18. $27.32

20. $32.12

22. $38.62

24. $34.15

21 Cash Register Calculations

2. 3 pennies, 3 quarters, 4 one dollar bills, 1 ten dollar bill

4. 2 quarters, 2 one dollar bills, 1 five dollar bill

6. 3 quarters, 3 one dollar bills, 1 ten dollar bill

8. 4 pennies, 1 nickel, 2 quarters, 1 five dollar bill, 1 ten dollar bill

10. 3 one dollar bills, 1 five dollar bill, 1 ten dollar bill, 1 twenty dollar bill

12. 1 penny, 1 nickel, 1 dime, 1 quarter, 3 one dollars, 1 five dollar

14. 2 dimes, 1 quarter, 1 one dollar, 1 five dollar, 1 ten dollar

16. 3 pennies, 1 nickel, 2 quarters, 1 one dollar, 1 five dollar, 4 twenty dollars

18. 1 penny, 1 one dollar, 1 ten dollar, 1 twenty dollar

20. 1 penny, 1 nickel, 2 quarters, 3 one dollars, 1 five dollar

22. 1 nickel

24. 2 pennies, 4 one dollars, 1 five dollar

26. 2 quarters

28. 1 penny, 1 nickel, 1 dime, 2 one dollars,

30. 1 nickel, 2 quarters, 1 one dollar, 1 ten dollar, 2 twenty dollars

22 Usual and Customary Prices

2. $17.20

4. $312.38

6. $5.47

8. $19.38

10. $78.91

12. $33.14

14. $5.56

16. $8.32

18. $5.62

20. $5.68

22. $16.10 (for 100)

24. $270.05

26. $4.78

28. $7.73

30. $11.30

32. $6.48

34. $7.13

36. $7.57

23 Discounts

2. $11.85

4. $85.41

6. $31.45

8. $166.35

10. $213.66

12. $112.77

14. $154.38

16. $355.96

18. $222.95

20. $469.20

22. $11.22

24. $80.91

26. $29.79

28. $157.59

30. $202.41

32. $128.51

34. $213.03

36. $134.12

38. $48.78

40. $108.03

24 Gross and Net Profits

2. $17.18, $11.18

4. $29.31, $23.31

6. $31.39, $25.39

8. $6.71, $0.71

10. $22.63, $16.63

12. $11.19, $7.19

14. $9.19, $5.19

16. $7.19, $3.19

18. $10.19, $6.19

20. $20.79, $15.79

22. $7.19, $3.19

24. $10.19, $6.19

26. $8.14, $4.14

28. $5.79, $1.79

30. $13.19, $9.19

25 Inventory Control

2. 8

4. 11

6. 1

8. 3

10. 4

12. 0

14. 4

16. 0

18. 2

20. 0

22. 0

24. 0

26. 0

28. 0

26 Daily Cash Report

2. Balance the following cash report:

	Reg 1	Reg 2	Reg 3	Total
+ Cash + Checks	1145.63		4322.12	5467.75
+ Bank Charges	366.12		980.35	1346.47
+ House Charges				
+ Paid Outs				
Total	1511.75		5302.47	6814.22
+ Closing Reading	354632.12		17524.82	372156.94
− Opening Reading	353099.50		12222.35	365321.85
= Difference	1532.62		5302.47	6835.09
− Coupons	18.90			18.90
− Discounts				
− Voids				
− Refunds				
− Over-rings				
Total	1513.72		5302.47	6816.19
+/−		−1.97	0	−1.97

4. Find the error in the
   following cash report, then
   balance the cash report:

	Reg 1	Reg 2	Reg 3	Total
+ Cash + Checks	1513.12	45.12	2002.02	3560.26
+ Bank Charges	120.00		350.44	470.44
+ House Charges				
+ Paid Outs				
Total	~~1393.12~~	45.12	2352.46	4030.70
	1633.12			
+ Closing Reading	105060.56	21012.12	210121.12	336193.80
– Opening Reading	103350.54	20967.00	207768.62	332086.16
= Difference	1710.02	45.12	2352.50	4107.64
– Coupons	1.10			1.10
– Discounts	8.90			8.90
– Voids	10.00			10.00
– Refunds				
– Over-rings	56.65			56.65
Total	1633.37	45.12	2352.50	4030.99
+/–	~~–210.25~~	0	–0.04	–0.29
	–0.25			

27 Parenteral Doses Using Ratio and Proportion Calculations

2. 2.4 ml

4. 0.5 L

6. 1 mg

8. 4.7 ml

10. 1.6 ml

12. 0.75 ml

14. 4 ml

16. 12.5 ml

18. 2 ml

20. 5 ml

22. 5 mls

24. 1 ml

26. 1.6 mls

28. 1.8 mls

30. 2.5 mls

32. 0.6 ml

34. 0.78 ml

36. 2 mls

38. 0.54 ml

40. 0.8 ml

28 Powdered Drug Preparations

2. 45 ml

4. 8 ml

6. 500,000 units/ml

8. 83.3 mg/ml

10. 11 ml

12. 200 mg/ml

14. 4 ml

16. 4.6 ml

18. 130 mg/ml

20. 18.4 ml

22. a) 0.2 ml

    b) 2.1 G

24. a) 3.6 mls

    b) 0.52 ml

26. 16.8 mls

28. a) 0.6 ml

    b) 0.8 ml

30. 1.25 mg/ml

32. 10.4 mls

34. 28.7 mls

36. a) 1 mg/ml

    b) 0.25 ml

38. 37.6 mls

40. 2 G/ml

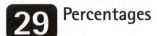 Percentages

2. 12%

4. 75 mg

6. 2.7%

8. 24 mg

10. 150 G

12. 12.5 G

14. 3.75 ml

16. 1500 mg

18. 4 ml

20. 37.5 ml

22. 80 G

24. 180 mg

26. 25 mls

28. 3.75 G

30. a) 7.02 G

   b) 234 mg/ml

32. 908 mg

34. 2.5 mls

36. 0.4%

38. 4% sulfamethoxazole

   0.8% trimethoprim

40. 45%

30 Ratio Solutions

2. 100 G

4. 1.5 G

6. 1.67%

---

8. 3.2 ml

10. 50 mg

12. 1:49

14. Lidocaine
200 mg;
epinephrine
0.2 mg

16. 2 mg

18. 25 mg

20. 1.2 ml

22. 10 mcg/ml

24. 0.5 ml

26. 1:12,500 w/v

28. 0.05%

30. a) 1:10,000 w/v

   b) 0.01%

32. 70 L

34. 0.02%

36. 500 mcg

38. 25 mls

40. 75 mg

31 Dosage Calculations Based on Body Weight

2. 2 tabs

4. 6 ml

6. 984 mg

8. 2 G

10. 83.3 ml

12. 3.5 ml

14. 0.825 G

16. 5 ml

18. 8 mg

---

20. .59 mg

22. 0.3 ml

24. 4.7 mls

26. 1.3 mls

28. 0.96 mls

30. 3.6 mls

32. 106.4 G

34. 4,128,960 units

36. 1.39 G

38. 27.3 mls

40. 37.2 mls

32 Dosage Calculations Based on Body Surface Area

2. 15 mg

4. 11.65 mg

6. 55 ml

8. 8.1 ml

10. 5.3 ml

12. 15.2 ml

14. 2 ml

16. 145 ml

18. 69 ml

20. 93.6 ml

22. 51.3 mls

24. 43.5 mls

26. 13.9 mls

28. 5.63 mls

30. 8.3 mls

32. 10.6 mls

34. 54 mls

36. 6.1 mls

38. 166.8 mls

40. 52.5 mls

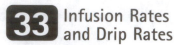 Infusion Rates and Drip Rates

2. 62.5 ml/hr

4. 3 bags

6. a. 10:00 p.m. 2200 Tuesday

   b. 2:30 a.m. 0230 Wednesday

   c. 7:00 p.m. 1900 Tuesday

   d. 10:00 a.m. 1000 Wednesday

8. 150 ml/hr

10. 30 ml/hr

12. 45 drops/min

14. 7 drops/min

16. 8hrs 20mins

18. 120 ml/hr

20. 300 ml

22. 1 hour 7 mins

24. 25 mins

26. 30 mins

28. 33 drops/min

30. 12:15 p.m.

32. 125 ml/hr

34. 120 mg

36. 10 bags

38. 150 ml/hr

40. 27 drops/min

34 Dilutions

2. 18.75%

4. 2%

6. 4.5%

8. 8 ml

10. Travasol 3.75%; dextrose 25%

12. 9.7%

14. 0.6%; 1:164

16. 72.3%

18. 4.4%

20. 64 ml

22. 1100 mls

24. 18 G ointment; 42 G petrolatum

26. 194 mls of a 50% solution

28. 2.88% Travasol and 23.08% dextrose

30. 1:710

32. 7.2 G ointment; 82.8 G petrolatum

34. 458.3 mls

36. 12 mls

38. 24 mls

40. 0.64%

35 Alligations

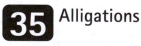

2. 444 ml of 50% and 3556 ml of 5%

4. 400 ml of 30% and 100 ml of 20%

6. 129 g of 10% and 321 g of 3%

8. 375 ml of 40% and 125 ml of water

10. 800 ml of 1:400 and 3200 ml of water

12. 1 ml

14. 167 ml of 70% and 833 ml of 40%

16. 1636 ml of 85% and 1364 ml of 30%

18. 80 ml of 80% and 400 ml of 8%

20. 3 fl. oz. of 10% and 1 fl. oz. of water

22. 1 L 31% and 1 L 27%

24. 86 mls stock solution and 34 mls water

26. 24 G 2.5 % ointment and 36 G petrolatum

28. 45 fl oz 20% and 19 fl oz water

30. 1000 mls 42% and 500 mls 18%

32. 231 mls 23.4% and 5769 mls water

34. 36 mls 8.4% and 14 mls 4.2%

36. 167 mls 60% and 83 mls water

38. 250 mls NS and 250 mls water

40. 14 mls NaCl and 986 mls water

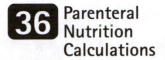

36 Parenteral Nutrition Calculations

	TPN No. 2	TPN No. 4
Sodium chloride	4.8 ml	8 ml
Potassium chloride	10 ml	7 ml
Magnesium sulfate	4.9 ml	4 ml
Potassium phosphate	3 ml	4 ml
Calcium gluconate	10 ml	51.6 ml
MVI	10 ml	10 ml
Trace elements	5 ml	5 ml
Vitamin C	4 ml	6 ml
Humulin R insulin	0.6 ml	0.95 ml
Folic acid	1 ml	0.75 ml
Sodium acetate	17.5 ml	7 ml
Potassium acetate	10 ml	4 ml
Sodium phosphate	5 ml	4 ml

6. 24 mls Sodium chloride
    25 mls Potassium chloride
    64.5 mls Calcium
    gluconate
    2.5 mls Magnesium sulfate
    6.7 mls Potassium
    Phosphate 2.4% Travasol
    and 5.7% Dextrose

8. 70 mls Potassium chloride
    42 mls Sodium chloride
    2 mls Magnesium sulfate
    20 mls Calcium gluconate
    3 mls Potassium phosphate
    6 mls Vitamin C
    3.92% Aminosyn
    25.1% Dextrose

NOTES

NOTES

NOTES

NOTES

NOTES